HARNESSING *the*
HEALING POWER
FRUIT *of*

HARNESSING *the*
HEALING POWER
FRUIT *of*

ROGER C. RINN, PhD
RALPH E. CARSON, PhD

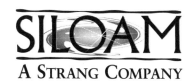

Most Strang Communications Book Group products are available at special quantity discounts for bulk purchase for sales promotions, premiums, fund-raising, and educational needs. For details, write Strang Communications Book Group, 600 Rinehart Road, Lake Mary, Florida 32746, or telephone (407) 333-0600.

Harnessing the Healing Power of Fruit
  by Roger C. Rinn, PhD, and Ralph E. Carson, PhD
Published by Siloam
A Strang Company
600 Rinehart Road
Lake Mary, Florida 32746
www.strangbookgroup.com

Scripture quotations marked niv are from the Holy Bible, New International Version. Copyright © 1973, 1978, 1984, International Bible Society. Used by permission.

Design Director: Bill Johnson
Cover design by Karen Gonsalves and Bill Johnson

Library of Congress Cataloging-in-Publication Data:
Rinn, Roger C.
  Harnessing the healing power of fruit / by Roger C. Rinn and Ralph E. Carson.
     p. cm.
  Includes bibliographical references.
  ISBN 978-1-59979-196-8
  1. Fruit--Therapeutic use. I. Carson, Ralph E. II. Title.
  RM237.R56 2009
  613.2'6--dc22
                              2009022160

This book was previously published by Rehoboth Publishing, LLC., copyright © 2008, ISBN 978-1-59979-487-7.

Neither the publisher nor the authors are engaged in rendering professional advice or services to the individual reader. The ideas, procedures, and suggestions in this book are not intended as a substitute for consulting with your physician. All matters regarding your health require medical supervision. Neither the authors nor the publisher shall be liable or responsible for any loss or damage allegedly arising from any information or suggestion in this book.

The recipes in this book are to be followed exactly as written. The publisher is not responsible for your specific health or allergy needs that may require medical supervision. The publisher is not responsible for any adverse reactions to the recipes contained in this book.

While the author has made every effort to provide accurate telephone numbers and Internet addresses at the time of publication, neither the publisher nor the authors assume any responsibility for errors or for changes that occur after publication.

09 10 11 12 13 — 9 8 7 6 5 4 3 2 1
Printed in Canada

To our grandkids

Aubrey Ellen Dithmer

Lily Morgan Dithmer

Richard William Rissmiller III

Acknowledgments

THERE ARE SO MANY PEOPLE INVOLVED IN BRINGING A PROJECT like this to fruition that it is impossible to name them all. We would, however, like to mention a few.

First, we thank our families for putting up with us during the research and writing of the book. Words can't express how much their love and support mean in our lives.

We thank our editors, designers, and typesetters for producing this book with its beautiful cover, interior design, and photo section. You made us look good!

Last but not least, we thank the team at Strang Communications for catching the vision of the importance of this message and making it possible for so many lives to be changed by reading it.

Contents

SECTION 1
Timeless Health Secrets for Today

SECTION 2
The Paradigm Shift From Treatment to Prevention

8 The Three Fs—Fiber, Fructose, and Fruit Juice 107

9 The Quest for Better Health 121

SECTION 3
Achieving Optimum Health

LIST OF ABBREVIATIONS

5LOX: 5-lipoxygenase

ACE: angiotensin-converting enzyme

AI: adequate intake

BMI: body mass index

CDC: Centers for Disease Control and Prevention

CO$_2$: carbon dioxide

COPD: chronic obstructive pulmonary disease

CRP: C-reactive protein

DASH: Dietary Approaches to Stop Hypertension

DRI: dietary reference intake

FDA: Food and Drug Administration

GST: glutathione-S-transferase

HCl: hydrochloric acid

HDL: high-density lipoprotein

HFCS: high-fructose corn syrup

HORAC: hydroxyl radical absorbance capacity

HPV: human papillomavirus

IOM: Institute of Medicine

IU: international unit

LDL: low-density lipoprotein

LFP: lychee fruit pericarp

NaCl: sodium chloride (table salt)

NCSH: National Center for Health Statistics

NHANES: National Health and Nutrition Examination Survey

NORAC: peroxynitrite radical absorbance capacity

OPC: oligomeric proanthocyanidin

ORAC: oxygen radical absorbance capacity

PAC: proanthocyanidin

ppm: parts per million

RDA: recommended daily allowance

RDI: recommended daily intake

ROS: reactive oxygen species

SOD: superoxide dismutase

S-ORAC: super-oxygen radical absorbance capacity

TAO: total antioxidant (assay)

TG: triglycerides

TIA: transient ischemic attack

UIL: upper intake level

USDA: United States Department of Agriculture

UTI: urinary tract infection

WHO: World Health Organization

FOREWORD

INALLY, A BOOK THAT REVEALS THE HEALING POWER OF FRUIT! Drs. Carson and Rinn have earned my deepest respect for their thorough and extensive work in the clinical field. They share my vision to challenge Americans to reclaim wellness, because it's inside each and every one of us. No matter what's going on in your life, you really can tap into that internal power and transform your life into one that really honors your dreams.

I've seen the health benefits of fruit firsthand in my own life and practice. Patients come to me desiring to be healthier but not knowing where to start. It's not enough just to say, "I want to lose thirty pounds" or "I want to get my blood pressure down." You have to know how each and every decision you make throughout the day can affect your health. That's where empowerment begins.

Over my years of advising patients, I've found that the best health-enhancing decisions we can make are often the simplest. By adding more fruits and vegetables to your diet, you can enhance the strength of your immune system and help lessen your risk for developing certain cancers. Studies have shown that the health properties of fruits such as blueberries and bilberries slow brain aging and maintain healthy vision.

These are just a few of the healing benefits of fruit. There are many, many more. I hope this helps you to understand why I am so excited about this book and how the knowledge within its pages will benefit so many people in extraordinary ways. This is a perfect resource for my patients who are ready to embrace a healthy lifestyle through better nutrition.

Every fruit product out there claims to be packed with health-promoting nutrients. But how do you know if the claims are true? Read this book carefully, and put the advice to work for you and your health!

—Andrea Pennington, MD, CAC
President, Pennington Empowerment Media
Author, *5 Steps to Total Wellness*

Introduction

S TAYING HEALTHY HAS BEEN AN OBSESSION FOR MODERN MEN AND women for centuries. Living longer, avoiding chronic illnesses, and being active and vibrant are the stuff of which dreams are made. Until recently, these have been merely pipe dreams and musings shared by humanity—hopes and yearnings with no paths to follow. No clearly defined prescription for success existed based upon scientific information or research. Over the past twenty-five years or so, a growing body of knowledge has emerged that has made these dreams of longevity and health more of a reality. There are now studies that suggest a path toward optimal health, increasing the probability of longer, healthier, and more active living.

The two of us have practiced our professions (Dr. Rinn is a psychologist and Dr. Carson is a nutritionist/exercise physiologist) for most of our adult lives. Our professions are focused on helping others. With the exciting developments in prevention, it was natural for us to pass on our findings to our patients. This book was the result of our commitment to helping others learn what we have discovered.

In this book, we will present the latest findings from food scientists and researchers on the beneficial aspects of consuming more fruits and fruit juices. We discuss the current crisis in dietary habits of Americans and how our dreadful eating patterns may create and exacerbate chronic illnesses. The evolving theory of inflammation will be outlined as one of the main driving forces for the development of deadly cancers, heart disease, and a plethora of other illnesses. The importance of fruits in performing anti-inflammatory services for the body will be demonstrated. Phytonutrients and their positive effects on your body's functioning will be detailed. Additional information about fruits and fruit juices will acquaint you with a vast array of findings helpful to maintaining your health and vigor.

Clearly, there are no guarantees in life except death and taxes. No human can expect to live forever on this earth. However, with up-to-date information and proper application of the data available in the scientific literature, it now appears possible to increase the probability of longer, healthier living. Consuming more fruit and fruit juices is one very important component of better health. The U.S. Department of Agriculture (USDA) has made the increase of fruits and fruit juices a primary concern of its educational efforts to get Americans leaner and healthier. Why it is so important to increase your fruit and fruit juice intake will become apparent as you read this book. Take responsibility for your health and the health of your loved ones now. Harness the benefits of fruits and fruit juices.

Timeless Health Secrets *for* Today

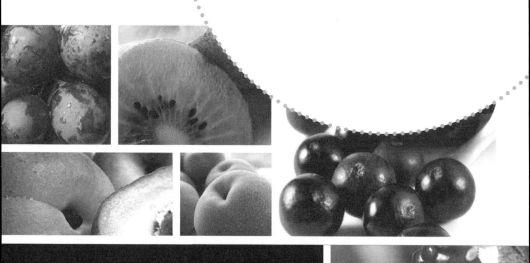

CHAPTER 1

TROUBLE *in* PARADISE

I F YOU ASK THE AVERAGE PERSON WHETHER PEOPLE IN THE UNITED States are living longer and have the best health-care system in the world, nine out of ten people will say yes.

However, according to many experts, including John Abramson, MD, a clinical instructor at Harvard Medical School, the United States ranks among the *worst*. In virtually every international comparison of health status, the United States is behind most other industrialized countries and even some of the third-world nations!

One of the most highly regarded of these measures is the World Health Organization's (WHO) "healthy life expectancy," a measure of total life expectancy minus years of illness. Among industrialized countries, the United States ranks an unbelievable 22, just two rankings ahead of the Czech Republic.[1]

This statistic exists in spite of the fact that we are No. 1 in health expenditures per capita. Each year more than $6,000 is spent on health care for every man, woman, and child in this country—more than twice as much as other developed countries spend.[2] Yet when the WHO takes these expenditures into account, America's health system's performance is ranked 37 among the nations of the world.[3] And when efficiency in improving citizens' health (meaning prevention methods) is added in, the United States drops to a dismal No. 72![4] In other words, we are paying the most to be among the worst! More people get cancer than ever before, and more people have diabetes and heart disease than ever before. Chronic fatigue and insomnia are more the norm than in the past, and more people suffer from depression and stress than ever before. This list could go on and on.

Why Are We Unhealthy?

Modern life brings negative forces that tend to undermine health efforts. In fact, many people you know—perhaps even you—face an uncertain health future as a result of today's fast-paced life, eating habits, and exercise habits.

Because of an abundance of food and modern lifestyle changes, Americans have steadily become more overweight and obese since the turn of the twentieth century and increasingly since the end of the Second World War.

Americans have been blessed with an ample food supply—lots of it. The problem with that food supply is that it has morphed into unhealthy foods to accommodate a fast-paced lifestyle. It's easier (and sometimes cheaper) to go through the local drive-through and order a double-stack greasy hamburger, hydrogenated oil–drenched fries, and a chemically laden soft drink. These convenient fast foods and prepared foods burden down current diets with high levels of added sugar and unhealthy fat.

As if nutritional habits weren't bad enough, add to that today's technology, such as television, text messaging, video games, computers, and the all-consuming World Wide Web, which keep people stuck in their seats and inactive. Eating comfort foods (pizzas, french fries, burgers, chips, soft drinks, doughnuts) while settling down on the couch in front of the TV has turned many of us into classic "couch potatoes."

And, unfortunately, as you will see in later chapters, these kinds of eating and exercise habits may cause many adults and, even worse, their kids, to become part of a chronically ill culture.

What We Eat and Drink Matters!

Remember your mom telling you to "eat your fruits and vegetables"? As a kid, you probably fought this tooth and nail, but you eventually did what you were told, biding your time until you were finally free of your mom's apron strings. Then, when you grew up, you ate what *you* wanted!

Greasy and sugary foods, quickly prepared and eaten on the run, have become meals of convenience and/or choice for many busy people. Does this sound familiar?

Sometimes we get dire warnings of the consequences during the dreaded annual physical examination (if we're smart enough to have one done) when the primary care physician discusses blood work results.

Many of us are momentarily shocked and frightened by the bad news, and we fervently promise the doctors and ourselves to mend our evil ways, eat more fruits and vegetables, stop snacking, quit drinking, exercise more, and lose weight—only to fall prey to that dreaded malady of life, *habit*. All too often, back we go to the bad old ways, and up go the bad cholesterol and body weight—while down go the chances of living a healthy and vibrant life.

Even the U.S. government has gotten in the fray. Most Americans have heard about the food pyramid, which has been around since the early 1990s as a simple device for recommending what to eat and about how much. But over the years, the food pyramid has been criticized as being inaccurate—with some even saying its real purpose was to create healthier pocketbooks for U.S. agribusinesses rather than a healthier population. In 2005, the USDA released a new and improved, customizable food pyramid called "MyPyramid." While most feel this new form of nutritional advice is an improvement over the original pyramid, some still find its recommendations debatable.

The Harvard School of Public Health suggests an alternative to the USDA food pyramid. The "Healthy Eating Pyramid," as they call it, is believed to follow the results of nutrition studies published in scientific journals more closely that the USDA pyramids.[5]

Be Honest: Has the Food Pyramid Helped Your Health?

If you're like most of our patients, you know about the food pyramid in one version or another, but you are only vaguely aware of the contents. And it shows!

Both the U.S. Department of Agriculture and the U.S. Department of Health and Human Services have long suggested that adults eat five fruits and vegetables a day. However, a 2005 study using self-reported dietary habits of Americans in all fifty states determined that only a third (32.6 percent) of all adults consumed two or more fruits on a daily basis, while less than a third (27.2 percent) ate three or more vegetables each day. In terms of eating habits, males, people with larger waistlines, and people under sixty-five years of age ate less fruits and vegetables than females, those over age sixty-five, or people who were not overweight. By the way, in this study, "fruit" referred to fruits *and* fruit juices, an important consideration in the diets of all.[6]

What can be learned from this research? It suggests that the mere presence of the food pyramid and the constant publishing and broadcasting of dietary guidelines are not enough to motivate over two-thirds of our population to eat better. And the news gets worse.

A study published by the U.S. Department of Agriculture makes the findings in the previous research even more depressing! The authors of the study found that when people were asked to estimate their consumption of fruits over a fourteen-day period, they actually ate "less fruit servings than they [thought] and much less than [was] recommended." For example, males ages twenty-five to fifty estimated they consumed 2.2 fruits daily while they actually ate only 0.9! Females ages twenty-five to fifty fared even slightly worse than their male counterparts, with an estimated consumption of 2.2 fruits daily but an actual level of 0.8 fruits actually eaten.[7]

So, the estimates by the USDA in that first study mentioned are undoubtedly even drearier than they already look. And we're doing even worse than we think! Just when you thought it was safe to eat five fruits and vegetables a day … *kaboom!*

The Department of Health and Human Services' Centers for Disease

Control and Prevention (CDC) combined forces with the Produce for Better Health Foundation and developed a program called "Fruits and Veggies—More Matters." In March 2007, the program was launched with a newer, more aggressive campaign to increase the consumption of fruits and vegetables even more.

Consumption guidelines have been published and now recommend *seven to thirteen* (count them, that is *not* a misprint!) servings of fruits and vegetables daily. So, in fact, when it comes to eating the optimal amount of recommended fruits and vegetables for good health, most people fall even shorter than they think!

An Important Word About Fruit Juices

When we mention the benefits of fruit juices in providing important antioxidants and phytonutrients and playing a significant role in disease prevention, we are talking about juices that contain the whole fruit—skin, pulp, and seed—and are minimally processed so that the juice contains live and active enzymes.

This does not apply to juices and juice drinks that have been pasteurized and clarified, watered down, or sweetened. For example, most apple, grape, and other fruit juices or juice drinks found in the grocery store are essentially sweetened water! These do not provide the benefits found in whole, minimally processed juices.

Why Are Fruits and Vegetables So Important for Your Health?

Get used to it. Live with it. Human beings really do need this higher level of fruits and vegetables—*seven to thirteen servings daily*—in their diets. Why?

Simply stated, we need more phytonutrients, antioxidants, vitamins, minerals, and fiber to combat chronic illnesses and aging. We will discuss these ideas in later chapters, but the basic idea is this: fruits, fruit juices, and vegetables help prevent many illnesses and unwanted conditions in large part because of their roles in producing antioxidants and helping control inflammation, which we also discuss later in this book.

Healthy Living in the Twenty-first Century

The twenty-first century is here, and it brings great news if you want to improve your family's health and enjoy a longer, healthier, and more vibrant life, no matter what your age! A new paradigm for healthy living has evolved over the past quarter century that puts the tools directly into your hands and lets you take charge.

Instead of waiting for diseases or chronic illnesses to strike and then relying on physicians to treat ailments, as your parents, grandparents, and all previous generations did, you now have options to prevent many of the most feared and difficult-to-treat health scourges that affect modern men and women.

In the twenty-first century, prevention isn't just the dream of centuries past; it is now a reality—and it's effective against many of the most dreaded diseases and debilitating health conditions, including heart disease, diabetes, osteoporosis, and even many cancers. While there are many incurable diseases, there are also many more that are curable. New discoveries and scientific breakthroughs and the increase in technological advances are helping people to live happier, healthier, longer lives. With early intervention and prevention, we can benefit from the greatest body of medical knowledge and the most sophisticated health care that has ever existed. Don't accept the *fait accompli*.

In the next chapter, we will see how sometimes inflammation is not necessarily bad. In fact, it's one of the most important defenses your body possesses to fight disease.

CHAPTER 2

INFLAMMATION—*the* BODY'S SWAT TEAM

INFLAMMATION. IT JUST SOUNDS BAD, BUT IT MAY SURPRISE YOU TO know that inflammation is one of the most important weapons in your body's health defenses.

How Inflammation Works

You are under constant bombardment every minute of your life by all sorts of unwanted, nasty, and potential disease-causing microbes. Inflammation, in essence, is your body's "SWAT team" that rushes to your defense and staves off attacks from the dangerous bacteria, viruses, and fungi that exist in your environment.

Inflammation—in the form of white blood cells and other substances from your immune system—is how your body is able to fight and defeat many of these potential invaders that threaten your health.

For example, when you cut your finger on an unseen nail—*ouch!*—your defenses quickly rush to protect you from bleeding to death immediately and/or dying from a subsequent systemic blood infection. If your protective system is working effectively, your blood starts clotting and any bacteria from the nail that managed to penetrate the skin are killed off by inflammation.

Then, in a few days, the wound is healed through several repair mechanisms, and the skin on your finger returns to its original condition, perhaps with a small scar remaining as a sign of the battle.

Acute vs. Chronic Inflammation

Acute inflammation

Early in the repair process, the area in and around an affected area, like the cut on your finger, typically gets red, is sensitive to touch, feels warm, and may swell somewhat. You may not be able move your finger at first. All perfectly normal—your finger is going through the *acute inflammation* stage, characterized by these five signs:

1. Heat

2. Loss of function

3. Pain

4. Redness

5. Swelling

"Acute" doesn't necessarily mean "severe"; however, it does refer to the quickness of the process and its short-term duration. In a typical injury like your cut finger, the acute inflammation protects the body for a few days while the blood forms clots and new tissue is built to return the skin to its protective role. When the inflammation is no longer necessary because the skin has been repaired, the acute inflammation ceases and—*voila!*—your finger is healed.

Chronic inflammation

Chronic inflammation is another thing altogether, when the inflammation process goes amok.

When inflammation becomes long-term and is either unnecessary or ineffective in defending against foreign invaders (i.e., viruses or bacteria), it is described as chronic, and it is harmful.

Unlike acute inflammation—which usually is beneficial—chronic inflammation is an unwanted and undesirable state in which the natural inflammatory processes work *against* the body. It causes damage to the tissues with changes in the cellular structure and dangerous scarring.

Of course, the body doesn't take this without a fight! Your defenses attempt to counteract the inflammation, often without success. If chronically inflamed areas of the human body are examined, white blood cells and other inflammatory substances such as macrophages (literally, big eaters) are often found in abundance as evidence. (Macrophages release free radicals, which cause cell and tissue damage leading to illnesses and aging. But more about macrophages later in the chapter.)

Unfortunately, much of the chronic inflammation in your body goes unnoticed—some health experts refer to it as "silent inflammation."

As you age, your body creates more inflammatory substances naturally and your anti-inflammatory responses become weakened. Scientists have shown that elderly persons who have become frail and disabled have significantly more inflammation in their bodies than those who are strong and active.[1]

Important

Chronic inflammation seems to be at the root of many of our serious illnesses and conditions.

To avoid premature aging and to maintain your vitality in your later years, controlling chronic inflammation is crucial. By working closely with your health-care provider, you can reduce chronic inflammation through a combination of traditional medicine and naturopathic alternatives such as changing your eating habits, exercising more, finding ways to reduce stress, and getting more rest.

In order to better understand how to reduce chronic inflammation, let's take a look at some of the causes.

What Causes Chronic Inflammation?

Genetics

Imagine yourself as a citizen of London or Genoa in the year 1450. The existence of germs was unknown. The hygiene of the era would have made a present-day health inspector run for the hills! Sewers were streams running down the streets. Wild dogs took care of garbage pickup. Infectious diseases ran amok, and shortly after delivery, many mothers and children died from "childbed fever." Most kids never made it to adulthood, and very few adults ever saw their fortieth birthday.

Presumably, the children and adults who had really aggressive, effective inflammatory responses to germs were the ones who primarily survived in those brutal times. And they passed on their aggressive inflammatory responses to their offspring.

Today, London, Genoa, and most of the civilized world do not have to cope with those terrible conditions. We are a germ-conscious society. We wash our hands with soap and water, physicians and midwives practice sterile techniques when delivering children, sewers are underground, and big trucks haul away our refuse. We are really clean. In fact, we are squeaky clean!

But our bodies' inflammatory responses haven't been able to turn on a dime along with the hygienic changes of modern society during the past several decades. Some scientists speculate that the robust inflammatory response developed throughout the centuries to help people survive to their forties now can be counterproductive and keeps many of us from living into our nineties or longer. Part of the answer to why we suffer from chronic inflammation, then, is in our own personal genetic makeup.

While we can't do anything about our genes, there's good news: many of the other sources of chronic inflammation are more or less under our control in most cases. Let's look at just a few.

Alcohol

Alcohol has been around for more than seven thousand years in Italy and the Middle East. In biblical days it was probably safer in the short run to drink beer and wine than to drink the germ-laden water!

Today, however, alcohol is one of the most common sources of chronic inflammation. Excessive drinking has been associated with an increase in:

- Cancer
- Heart problems
- Liver and pancreatic disease
- And many other undesirable outcomes

Recent research indicates that red wine and other alcoholic beverages contain antioxidants, which in *moderate* amounts may be "good" for the body.

But what is considered "moderate?" The safest levels are different for men and women, as recommended by the U.S. Department of Agriculture in their Dietary Guidelines for Americans—2005.[2]

- Men should keep their intakes at no more than two drinks daily.

- Women should have not more than one drink daily.

- A "drink" is defined as a 12-ounce bottle of regular beer, a 5-ounce glass of wine, or 1½ ounces of 80 percent proof distilled spirits (gin, vodka, bourbon)

NOTE: These guidelines do not suggest *daily* drinking. What they suggest is that alcohol is a potential source of inflammation, which is something *you can* control. If you do drink, keep your intake well within the suggested levels. If you don't drink, now is not the time to start.

Cholesterol

Cholesterol has a bad reputation, but, in fact, it is important for tissue functioning and repair and for several important chemical reactions in the body.

Cholesterol is carried in the blood inside spherical structures called lipoproteins. There are two types of lipoprotein—low-density (LDL) or high-density (HDL). Low-density lipoprotein (LDL) is most often referred to as "bad" cholesterol, taking cholesterol to the cells. LDL is associated with increased inflammation. High-density lipoprotein (HDL) is often referred to as "good" cholesterol, helping to take excess cholesterol from the cells to the liver. HDL appears to be anti-inflammatory.

Most cholesterol is manufactured in your body's organs such as the liver, the intestines, and other organs. Some is provided by what you eat—with certain foods contributing to higher levels of cholesterol.

When (and if) you go to see your doctor for an annual physical, the doctor will send you for blood tests to check the various levels in your body, including your cholesterol levels. Think of that test as the doctor's "lie detector": if you think about lying (or fibbing) about your nutrition and lifestyle habits, this test will reveal the truth. Diet is intimately associated with cholesterol levels. The more you eat, the lower the percentage of cholesterol, which is naturally manufactured by your body. *Therefore, if you eat more food, what you eat has greater effects on your health, good or bad.*

And it's not only the *quantity* of food you eat, but it's also the *quality* of the food. If you eat lots of red meat, cook with vegetable oils (some are OK), and eat other inflammation-inducing foods that have higher LDL levels (bad cholesterol), eventually it will catch up to you in the form of more inflammation. If you eat more fruits and vegetables, you have a greater chance of lowering your LDL levels and reducing inflammation.

Understanding Cholesterol Levels

For normal adults with no significant risk factors or illness, total cholesterol below 200 is probably sufficient.

Even if you are doing all the right things to lower your LDL cholesterol levels, your doctor may still need to find a treatment to control it. Usually it is a result of your genetic makeup, and, as we said earlier, there's nothing you can do about that. But take heart—you can overcome it if you follow your doctor's advice and continue to follow a program of eating healthy and exercising.

Infections

Sometimes chronic inflammation is a result of chronic infections in the body. Think of it as your body being under constant attack and constantly in defense mode to protect itself from foreign invaders.

When you have a virus or bacteria in your body, an infection will prompt your body to mobilize its defensive armaments. Occasionally, your white blood cells and other weapons are not sufficient to kill the infectious invaders. Too many white cells over a long a period of time cause chronic inflammation.

For example, many years ago when we were in graduate school, ulcers were thought to be caused by stress and worry. We now know that most ulcers are caused by bacteria in the stomach, called *helicobacter pylori*, which can cause chronic infection. After years of "war" between these bacteria and our own white blood cells (which results in chronic inflammation), ulcers are formed, and occasionally cancer develops.

The same inflammatory process appears to occur when a woman becomes infected with the *human papillomavirus (HPV)*, known years ago to cause "venereal warts." After many years of this chronic irritation of the cervix, cervical cancer may ensue.

Obesity and fat-distribution patterns

We all have fatty tissue—and, in fact, a certain amount of fat is necessary for the human body to function properly. In general, recommended levels of body fat are about 15–18 percent for men and 22–25 percent for women. Many of us are well over this necessary level! Obesity is now reaching epidemic proportions. Approximately 65 percent of the adult population in the United States is obese, which may cause them to experience chronic health problems in the future due to obesity.[3]

Many obese people are extremely overweight because of poor eating habits and lack of exercise. If they continue to eat foods that are high in fat, sugar, and salt, eventually the body will produce a buildup of plaque in the heart, leading to heart disease.

Are You an Android or a Gynoid?

No, we're not referring to extraterrestrials; we're referring to fat distribution. Too much body fat is dangerous. Here's a quick (and shocking!) rule of thumb: the heavier you are relative to your height, the more inflammation your body's fat will produce.

There are two common forms of fat distribution in human bodies: android and gynoid.

- *Android* fat distribution pattern centers in and on the abdomen; i.e., the classic "beer belly."

- *Gynoid* fat distribution is carried mostly in the buttocks, hips, and thighs.

Of the two, android fat is the most problematic. Why? The fatty tissue we see is not all on the surface, but it often surrounds the organs of our gut such as the stomach, colon, and pancreas. Processes in fatty tissue cause white blood cells and other inflammatory substances to focus particularly on areas of fatty deposits in the abdomen. These organs are then bombarded by chronic inflammation.

The body mass index (BMI)

The body mass index (BMI) was developed to take into account the height and weight of an individual when determining whether the person is at risk for chronic illnesses. Generally speaking, the more you weigh in comparison to your height, the closer you are to obese, which puts you at risk for many serious illnesses.

A person who weighs 175 pounds and is six feet tall is not considered obese. However, if a person weighs 175 pounds and is five feet tall, that person would be classified obese and is at greater risk for many illnesses.

How to Compute Your BMI

Multiply your weight in pounds by 703.
Then divide by your height in inches squared.
Then compare with the table below to see where you fall.

BMI	Classification
Less than 18.5	Underweight
18.5–24.9	Normal
25.0–29.9	Overweight
30.0–39.9	Obese
40.0+	Morbidly obese

For optimal health, keep your BMI in the range of normal. If you are above 24.9, get that excess weight off now.

Other sources of chronic inflammation

There are other sources of chronic inflammation in our lives, too many to detail in this book. However, a partial list should suffice in letting you know that inflammation has many causes.

Some of these are less in your control than others—for example, air pollution—*but most are sources over which you have significant control:*

- Air pollution (living in large urban areas with many automobiles and trucks)

- Diabetes (particularly if you do not monitor your blood sugar and treat the disorder appropriately)

- Hot beverages

- Salty foods

- Sleep deprivation (getting less than eight hours nightly)

- Stress, including chronic anxiety, depression, hostility, and insomnia

- Stomach acid (which can be propelled up into the lower part of the esophagus—gastroesophageal reflux disease—and results in "heartburn," changes in cell structure, and potentially cancer)

- Tobacco products (smoked or chewed)

You should be getting more familiar with these, as many are the same as the modifiable risk factors for cancer.

- Overweight/obesity (particularly abdominal fat)

- Drinking alcohol in excess (see guidelines we mentioned earlier)

- High blood pressure

- Cholesterol (high LDL and low HDL)

- Periodontal disease (bacteria in the gums)

- High homocysteine (caused by low levels of vitamins B_2, B_6, B_{12}, and folic acid)

- Physical inactivity

Do you notice a pattern? It should be coming through loud and clear! By now, you should have some understanding about chronic inflammation and why controlling it is so important in maintaining your health.

Chronic Inflammation and Your Body

Chronic inflammation and pro-inflammatory cytokines

Macrophages are one of the first lines of defense that try to eat or engulf the invader; for example, a bacterium. (Remember, this process starts producing free radicals as a result of oxidation.)

At the same time, signaling cells send out the SOS to white blood cells and others for help. These signaling cells are called *pro-inflammatory cytokines.* Cytokines let the body know that invaders are present and that help is needed.

The presence of these pro-inflammatory cytokines can be measured in your blood supply and let your health-care provider know that inflammation is present in the body.

Some of the more common inflammation-signaling cytokines have biochemical names you may have heard of, including tumor necrosis factor-alpha, interleukin 1, and interleukin 6.

Chronic inflammation and C-reactive protein (CRP)

In 1930, two researchers, William S. Tillett and Thomas Francis Jr., identified a substance in the blood of individuals with acute inflammation, which they called C-reactive protein (CRP). It was later discovered that a rise in CRP was correlated with interleukin 6, the pro-inflammatory cytokine mentioned above.

CRP has been used as a very general, nonspecific marker of inflammation for many years. We all manufacture this substance in our livers. Some of us inherit higher levels of CRP than others do.

However, individuals who smoke, have high blood pressure, suffer from colon cancer, are overweight, or lead sedentary lives tend to have higher CRPs. Individuals prone to strokes and heart attacks appear to have higher CRPs.

Conversely, thin individuals who are physically active (and presumably have more fruits in their diets) have lower CRPs and appear to have lowered risks of cardiovascular disease.*

Your health-care provider can check your CRP with a simple, inexpensive blood test (usually by requesting high-sensitivity C-reactive protein, [hs CRP]). Knowing your CRP may motivate you to either lower it or keep it low.

---

* See P. M. Ridker, "Clinical Application of C-Reactive Protein for Cardiovascular Disease Detection and Prevention," *Circulation* 107 (2003): 363–369, for a review of CRP.

Chronic inflammation and cancer

Of all modern diseases, cancer is probably the most feared. Despite the advances in science and health care in general, too many suffer from its ravages or die every year.

Cancer occurs when cells in our bodies begin to grow and divide without limits. Normal tissue tends to stay where it belongs, but not cancerous tissue. It tends to invade nearby structures in our bodies and may begin to grow in areas far from the original site (metastatic cancer). Depending upon what stage the cancer has reached, treatment may be long and painful.

Cancer risk factors

There are two main ways in which we might develop cancer. First, we can inherit the probability of getting the disease through our DNA. For example, about 10 percent of all women with breast cancer have an abnormal gene that is associated with the development of the malignancy.[4]

Second, we can develop the disease via environmental factors leading to chronic inflammation, which in turn seems to alter our DNA. The sources of this inflammation can include chronic infections from viruses or bacteria and chronic irritations from mechanical or chemical sources. Examples include bacteria such as *helicobacter pyloris* and the human papillomavirus (HPV) as inflammation "factories" that increase the probability of cancer. Tobacco and its products are among the leading chemical causes of many cancers, including lung and colon cancer. Air pollution is yet another. Mechanical causes may include the continuous contact of an ill-fitting dental appliance (such as a bridge) against the inside of one's mouth, resulting in chronically inflamed tissue.

Modifiable risk factors for cancer

The respected and venerable British medical journal *The Lancet* published a very important article that goes to the heart of inflammation and cancer, suggesting that there are nine modifiable risk factors under your control that are associated with the development of 35 percent of all cancers.[5]

Nine Modifiable Risk Factors for Cancer (in order of importance)

1. Smoking (tobacco)

2. Alcohol to excess (beer, wine, and distilled spirits)

3. *Low intake of fruits and vegetables* (our emphasis)

4. Overweight/obesity

5. Physical inactivity

6. Unsafe sex (specifically, contracting HPV)

7. Urban air pollution

8. Indoor smoke from household fuels

9. Contaminated injections in health-care settings

By altering your lifestyle, you should be able to reduce your personal risk of developing cancer by more than one-third.

And for certain diseases, you can lower your risk even more. For example, you can raise your chances of avoiding esophageal cancer by 85 percent; mouth and oropharynx cancer by 80 percent; trachea, bronchus, and lung cancer by 87 percent; and cervix uteri cancer by 100 percent![6]

These findings are extremely important, and all point to the influence of reducing sources of chronic inflammation that contribute to cancer. Of particular interest in this book is the finding that consuming more fruits, fruit juices, and vegetables reduces our chances of developing cancer.

The conclusion reached is that a variety of highly pigmented fruit helps prevent cancer. However, you cannot say oranges, blueberries, mangoes, or any other fruit for that matter prevents cancer.

Extensive review of scientific literature has demonstrated that there is evidence for protective effect from plant fruits in the diet. The American Institute of Cancer Research recommends basing all meals on plant food due to research findings that show a diet including vegetables and fruits may protect against cancer.[7] Much of the research supports that fruits contain many different types and amounts of phytochemicals. For example, one orange may contain up to sixty known anticancer phytochemicals.

Researchers believe that the optimal benefit would come from eating whole fruits, but recent reports suggest that fruit juice is also beneficial. A review of eleven studies concluded that the cancer and cardiovascular benefits may be more attributable to antioxidants rather than fiber.[8] The view that pure fruit juices are nutritionally inferior to fruit in relation to chronic disease risk is not justified.

Chronic inflammation and heart disease

Heart attack is the No. 1 killer among men and women around the world. Like cancer, many heart attacks are preventable. The most common type of heart attack is called a myocardial infarction. Myocardial infarction occurs when the blood supply to the heart muscle (the myocardium) is blocked (infarcted) by a blood clot (thrombus) and some of the heart muscle dies (becomes necrotic) as a result of the interrupted blood and oxygen flow (ischemia).

How does this happen? Many years of chronic inflammation from excessive LDL ("bad" cholesterol) and triglycerides cause a buildup of atheromatous plaques (literally, "a lump of porridge" in Greek). These deposits on the sides of the arteries cause the opening for blood flow (the lumen) to narrow (stenosis). When a piece of the plaque breaks off, it forms a clot (thrombus). If the clot is "upstream" from a significantly narrowed area and is sufficiently large, it will plug the smaller opening of an occluded vessel, and a heart attack ensues.

Exactly the same process occurs in so-called ischemic strokes. (Hemorrhagic strokes are the result of vessels rupturing and bleeding, which are less under our control.) With strokes, the blood supply is cut off to the brain.

While not everyone has the same experience, here are some common signs of a heart attack and a stroke:[9]

Heart attack	Stroke
Chest pain or discomfort (uncomfortable pressure, squeezing)	Sudden weakness or numbness in the face or limbs
Upper body discomfort in one or both arms, back, neck, jaw, or stomach	Trouble speaking and understanding
Shortness of breath	Dizziness or loss of balance
Nausea, vomiting, light-headedness, or breaking out in a cold sweat	Sudden, severe headache with no known cause

In both heart attacks and strokes, tissue begins to die quickly, so time is always of the essence. Get help immediately if you think you are having a stroke or heart attack. *However, it is infinitely better to avoid these problems in the first place.*

Two related disorders of the cardiovascular system are angina pectoris (often referred to as angina) and transient ischemic attack (often called TIA, or ministroke). Angina is a brief heart episode in which the heart muscle is deprived of oxygen due to the narrowing of an artery supplying blood to the heart, caused by a temporary blockage or spasm of the vessel. The angina sufferer can experience anything from chest discomfort to excruciating pain.

A TIA is a similar disorder of the arteries supplying the brain and may mimic an actual stroke in everything but duration. Both of these conditions are warning signs of serious underlying arterial problems, are associated with future heart attacks or strokes, and require immediate medical attention.

If you're reading carefully, you'll note that all of the risk factors for heart attack appear to be associated with inflammation. The obvious prescription for avoiding a heart attack lies in the careful pursuit of good health habits!

Diet is one of the most potent interventions for prevention of that first or second heart attack. Drastically reduce your intake of saturated fats, eat more deep-sea fish (like salmon) for more omega-3 fatty acids, and increase your intake of fruits and vegetables.

Those whose diets included the highest fruit intake had more than 70 percent reduced risk of heart problems than those who ate the least amount of fruit. On average, for every additional piece of fruit consumed each day, subjects showed a 10 percent reduction in coronary risk.[10]

Risk Factors for Heart Attacks

The risk factors for heart attacks are numerous. There is really nothing that you can do about a few of them. These include:

- Being older than sixty

- Being male

- Having a hereditary predisposition (a blood relative with a history of heart disease)

You can't change the above risk factors. What *does* work is paying attention to the factors you *can* modify to lower your chances of having a myocardial infarction.

Now that we have a basic understanding of how chronic inflammation affects the body, let's take look at how reducing inflammation and the risks associated with it can help bring the body back into homeostasis—back into balance.

CHAPTER 3

BRINGING *the* BODY INTO BALANCE

EXCEPT FOR ANTIBIOTIC TREATMENTS AND CHEMOTHERAPY, FEW other medications produce a cure for illnesses. Does that statement surprise you? We consume billions of dollars of pharmaceuticals annually, both prescription and over the counter. Without question, those pills, injections, patches, and liquids are important to our comfort, survival, ability to function, and longevity, but they usually don't cure anything. Indeed, the body heals itself. Sometimes the medicines we use give our bodies time to heal, act as a catalyst for (encourage) healing, lower the risk of getting a disease, or reduce the symptoms of the disease, but they do not do the healing work—our bodies do that. And the key to the healing mechanism is homeostasis.

Homeostasis is the tendency of your body to seek and maintain equilibrium. Inherent in this definition is the concept of balance. If your temperature increases above its normal level of 98.6 degrees Fahrenheit (more or less), mechanisms in your body engage to lower the temperature. If your temperature decreases below an optimal level, other mechanisms make their appearance to raise your temperature back to 98.6. In healthy individuals, if you eat too much at one meal, you are not as hungry at the next. If you skip a meal, you may eat more the next. Health is developed and maintained when you have a balance in your whole body's functioning, or homeostasis. Diseases occur when your equilibrium is disturbed, when the body is out of balance.

A Cultural View

The notion of homeostasis is nothing new and can be traced to earlier civilizations such as China, India, and the Navajos, among others. The Navajos believed that the goal of life was to live in harmony with one's entire environment and called this process *hozho*. Modern man typically will dam a river to avoid flooding, fighting with and conquering the elements. Hozho would lead man simply to move out of a flood plain. Harmony and balance were practiced in all aspects of life, leading the Navajo to "go with the flow," so to speak. Along with this attitude, good and evil were considered as complementary. One could not exist without the other. We cannot even think about good without implying its opposite. Each needs the other. Harmony and balance were at the core of this belief.

Harmony within one's self has long been sought by practitioners of yoga. The word *yoga* is from the Sanskrit meaning "to join" or "to yoke." This relates to the yoga objective of joining mind, body, and spirit. The underlying premise of yoga is the fusion of these three entities via respect, kindness, and compassion. Those practicing yoga use a combination of mindful exercises including postures (asanas), controlled breathing (pranayama), and meditation. It follows that such techniques were aimed at "yoking" together the mind, body, and spirit to produce harmony and balance.

Traditional Chinese medicine focuses very particularly on homeostasis through the concepts of yin and yang. The universe and our bodies are conceptualized as collections of opposites like sunlight and shade, hot and cold, acidic and basic. Yin is viewed as expanding, cold, wet, slow, passive, sweet, loose, and dark. Yang is contracting, hot, dry, fast, aggressive, salty, tight, and light. Disease occurs when there is imbalance in the body, and health is the result of equilibrium. Both yin and yang are important to our body's health and must be in balance according to the precepts of Chinese medicine.

Central to traditional Chinese medicine is food. The Chinese viewed food in four distinct ways. First, there was food as diet. This concept meant that food provided the necessary substances for life, growth, and health. Second, food as tonic referred to the use of food to treat individuals who were experiencing general weakness with no specific disease. A tonic might be used when someone had been ill and was recovering and needed strength. Third, food as medicine meant its use to treat imbalances that had led to diseases. In this sense, food was the treatment. Finally, the fourth concept was food as abstention, referred to as the practice of avoiding foods that could create an imbalance and thus an illness. From the yin and yang, the field of macrobiotics was born out of teachings of the ancients, the Tao.

Macrobiotics is a way of living that purportedly places us in harmony with the natural order of the universe. Not only does it refer to food as diet, but it is also concerned with the natural order of the universe and is a spiritual approach to living. Vegetables and whole grains, according to macrobiotics, have the most balanced energies and create "peaceful energy" within us. As we have seen earlier, yin and yang are opposites; in macrobiotics, yin is seen as the tendency of a food to disperse and yang the tendency of a food to gather. For example, thinking of dietary minerals, yin represents foods rich in potassium, and yang represents foods rich in sodium. Brown rice has both potassium and sodium, so it is thought to be a relatively balanced food. If we eat foods too high in yin, we may experience fatigue and a lack of focus; too high in yang, we may experience anxiety. The practitioner of traditional Chinese medicine may prescribe a combination of foods and seasonings appropriate for each season (no pun intended) of the year.

The mere fact that diverse cultures have a place for the notion of balance—homeostasis—in their beliefs and rituals suggests that the concept bears a closer look. Does this relate to real people in the twenty-first century?

The Human Body

How does homeostasis relate to your body and health? As we noted earlier, the natural mechanisms of the body force a return to balance when something is out of sync. For example, your blood maintains an optimum pH (alkalinity/acidity) of 7.4. A slight change in this value either up or down can cause havoc in the body. Once the body senses this change of acidity, its entire system cranks into action to return the pH to 7.4.

Cholesterol is another physiological entity that relates directly to health issues and is subject to homeostasis. Too much of the "bad cholesterol" (LDL) in the blood causes blood vessels to become clogged; too little results in excessive bleeding. A complex feedback system in the liver controls the amount of "good" and "bad" cholesterol available to the cells, within limits.

Genetics and diet can push the system out of balance, as we covered in the last chapter. Then, disease makes its appearance. We constantly hear about high blood pressure and know it can lead to vascular disease, kidney failure, strokes, and heart attacks. Low blood pressure is equally dangerous, ultimately causing debilitation and occasionally death if untreated. The blood vessels either contract or dilate to control pressure, again within limits. Calcium levels are kept at constant concentration in the blood. If there is too little, the body leaches calcium from the bones, and the result is osteoporosis. If there is too much, the result can be kidney stones and hardening of the arteries. Again, the body works very hard to keep everything in balance—homeostatic.

Even exercise succumbs to the need for balance. Too much exercise and your cortisol system breaks down the very muscles you are endeavoring to develop. Too little exercise and your muscles atrophy. There is an old saying among fitness gurus: "That which is used develops, and that which is not, wastes away." Indeed, exercise has several dimensions: strength, endurance, and flexibility. A person can be very strong from lifting weights but have no endurance or flexibility. Our conditioning should include all three of these attributes in balance. If you do not exercise competing muscle groups around a joint, for instance, problems can result, including sprains, arthritis, bursitis, tendonitis, and other injury. Equilibrium is the name of the game.

This book is about food. Nothing is more pertinent to health maintenance than the concept of a *balanced diet*. At the heart of the balanced diet are the fifty-five or so essential nutrients thought to be necessary for maintenance, growth, and repair of the body. Nutrients are called "essential" if the body does not manufacture them. The body is totally dependent upon food to supply these *essential nutrients*. To ensure that you are getting all the necessary proteins, vitamins, and minerals essential to life, you only need to consume minimum amounts from the four basic food groups: *fruits and vegetables* for vitamin A, vitamin C, folic acid, potassium, and trace minerals; *eggs and fish* for protein, vitamin B_{12}, vitamin B_6, zinc, and iron; *dairy* for calcium and minerals; and *starches and grains* for other B vitamins and minerals. Fiber is not an essential nutrient despite its importance to long-term health. This will be discussed in detail in a later chapter.

Many years ago, wealthy customers of grain mills were given refined flour, pure white in color, and absent of vitamin B_1 as a result of the process. Those unlucky users of the beautiful white product often suffered from beriberi because the vitamin was missing. A vegetarian can comfortably and safely exist without the use of animal products (eggs, fish, and meat) by obtaining protein from vegetable sources. However, vegetarians need to supplement their diets with vitamin B_{12} and monitor their intakes of iron and zinc. Supplements can serve as a viable source of calcium. Not only is balance about obtaining enough essential nutrients to survive, but it can also be about not getting too much of any one item. Excess meat can create significant health problems due to too much fat or too much protein, putting stress on the liver and kidneys.

Neurobiology and Behavior

The human brain is likewise designed with opposing functions. It is wired to seek pleasure and avoid pain. The brain possesses areas that support the "feel-good" function, including structures such as the nucleus accumbens and the left prefrontal cortex with the neurotransmitters dopamine and serotonin. It also has areas that are vigilant for danger and pain and produce anxiety—the amygdala and the right prefrontal cortex with the neurotransmitter norepinephrine. Ideally, your brain assists you in seeking and obtaining pleasure without allowing you to take too great a risk in the process. This helps you ride your bicycle downhill at a good, exhilarating clip, but, hopefully, at the point of unsafe speed, you put on the brakes.

This balancing act of brain functions may be seen in the development of depression. Why would the human species develop depression? When an animal is trapped by prey (thus preventing flight) and is not strong enough to actively defend itself (eliminating the fight option), it often freezes, a complete inhibition of action called *learned helplessness* by psychologist Martin Seligman.[1] The act of freezing by the helpless animal may be quite useful in its overall survival, avoiding potentially lethal fights with larger or more aggressive beasts. Dr. Seligman and his colleagues have cataloged a number of ways helplessness in animals and depression in humans seem to parallel one another. Although it is beyond the scope of this book to discuss the myriad ways in which helplessness and depression are very similar, suffice it to say that helplessness is a common explanation for depression among many mental health professionals.[2]

Depression in humans may often be preceded by events that are (perceived or actually) out of the sufferer's control, leading to a loss of self-confidence and thus helplessness. After a series of such events and in the absence of skills to flee or fight, the individual may become depressed. Depression may have an upside even today, since some behavioral research suggests that depressed individuals are often rewarded for their symptoms and behaviors. Others often take over tasks not being completed by their sad loved ones, treat them with kid gloves, and pamper them. A happy partner or relative is expected to pitch in. Notice the presence of balance once again.

Our brain possesses a number of structures comprising the emotional functions of humans, namely the *limbic system*. Again, the tendency of our bodies to seek and find homeostasis is amazing. Lower primates such as monkeys rely on their emotional center to cope with stressful situations. Take a group of monkeys and subject them to a predator from which there is no escape, clearly a stressful circumstance. Most if not all of these little fellows will behave in an instinctive, stereotypical manner, gesturing (often referred to as posturing in humans) by screaming, jumping up and down, and baring their teeth in an effort to frighten the intruder. When this tactic is unsuccessful, they resort to grooming (often referred to as self-soothing). Grooming involves the removal of tiny parasites from their fur and eating them, a pleasurable experience to which they return repeatedly in times of stress. When they mate, monkeys appear to be attacking each other. This ritual is completed by mutual grooming, each participating in calming the other. Mother monkeys do the same to their babies, grooming them in times of stress. We are not much different.

Imagine you are happily filling out your federal tax return, expecting a refund. At the bottom of the page, you discover you owe Uncle Sam five thousand dollars. You may head for the refrigerator and grab a candy bar or some other so-called "comfort food." The unpleasant and unexpected experience (pain) of funding Congress's coffers is countered by the sweet, creamy, and chocolate flavor of a bar (pleasure). This is homeostasis at its best.

You can see that the brain functions to maintain homeostasis in humans. If you perceive a crisis or negative event, you will experience discomfort (e.g., fear, anger, sadness, and boredom) and will ultimately attempt to balance this pain with something pleasurable. This pattern is readily seen in people who struggle with addictions and other maladaptive behaviors. Individuals dependent upon alcohol enter a recovery program and are often successfully abstinent after treatment, a rather uncomfortable state initially. What do many recovering individuals turn to instead of alcohol when under stress? Right, they turn to food. A person dependent upon tobacco stops smoking. What do these individuals turn to instead of tobacco? Right again, food. Now for the bonus question: What do dieters turn to when they successfully lower their intake of food? Right again! The dieters frequently will "tough it out" and experience a horribly uncomfortable empty feeling, a veritable void (pain), suffering until at last…too much and inappropriate food intake is replaced in the repertoires of the dieters' behaviors (pleasure). Once weight has been regained and the pre-diet weight often surpassed, guilt and self-condemnation are experienced (pain) and the cycle is repeated. Most diets end in failure. This may help explain such dismal outcomes of most diets. Moreover, occasionally the dieter is so overcome with the pain of low calorie intake that the pleasure of eating creates a feeling of extreme ecstasy, perhaps resulting in binge eating. Sometimes an individual feels that life is out of control (pain). Dieting is control (pleasure), and successful dieting (losing large amounts of weight) is ultimate control, resulting in anorexia nervosa, which is another topic altogether.

We could go on and on about the balance of behavior, which is not the focus in this chapter. There are nutritional discoveries and developments that help bring the body into a state of homeostasis, namely antioxidants and phytonutrients.

The Antioxidant Revolution

One exciting and popular nutritional development over the last twenty-five years has been the findings surrounding *antioxidants* and their contributions to health and longevity. What we in the West view as a healthy nutritional program is based upon principles and myths that have endured countless changes in government policy, naturopathic ideology, consumer scrutiny, public fickleness, and folklore. Nonetheless, the notions of variety, balance, and moderation have survived the test of time and the ever-changing landscape of "more is better" and "the latest miracle supplement." Antioxidants are one purported "miracle." Often we are unduly impressed by claims that a particular product has the largest quantity of vitamin C in its class, the most efficiently absorbed mineral, the greatest concentration of a particular antioxidant, or the highest ORAC (oxygen radical absorbance capacity) score. (We will take a closer look at the ORAC score in chapter 6.)

As in all areas of life, having the most of a particular commodity (e.g., land, money) does not guarantee happiness or health. You know that if the capacity of a cup is 8 ounces, trying to fill it with 10 ounces is a waste. The cup can only hold so much. It does not get "fuller" or "better" just because it is provided with more than its capacity. The body operates in the same manner. Giving an athlete a huge quantity of protein to bulk up makes absolutely no sense if there are not enough carbohydrates with which to build muscle. If a supplement contains a large amount of beta-carotene, an excess will block the absorption of other valuable carotenes: remember, the cup can only hold so much. Why take a large dosage of pycnogenol to prevent cancer if too much may allow cancer cells already present in the body to survive, multiply, and spread? Why take L-carnitine if your body already produces all it needs? More is not always better. There is indeed too much of a good thing.

How much of a nutrient does the body need?

There are certainly extremes between too much, when the amount is toxic to life, and too little, when the amount results in illness or death. In the middle range between deficiency and toxicity lies a wide range of intakes that support health—to varying degrees. In the past, nutrient needs were determined by the level needed to cure a deficiency's symptoms. If the absence of a nutrient resulted in an illness, it was deemed *essential.* The deficiency of vitamin C resulted in scurvy, a debilitating disease suffered by British sailors in the days of Sir Francis Drake and others. Limes, which contain ample vitamin C, were given to the sailors, and the disease was successfully treated; thus, British sailors were referred to as "Limeys." Today, nutrient needs are determined by the amount of a particular nutrient needed to support *optimal health.* Although the amount of vitamin C needed to successfully treat scurvy is relatively small, the amount thought to reduce the risk of some cancers is much larger. Furthermore, nutrients are being examined in the context of the whole diet. Health benefits are not limited to vitamin C, but also include those fruits and vegetables rich in vitamin C, which also provide many other nutrients and non-nutrients (such as phytochemicals), all important for optimal health. Undoubtedly, antioxidants are important, but they are merely part of the armamentarium of healthy living. We will revisit them in a later chapter. As exciting as the antioxidant findings are to understanding the origins of chronic illnesses, we have now entered a new era even more promising for preventive medicine—inflammation.

Inflammation: A New Paradigm in Prevention

Without question, those of us in the modern, industrialized nations have benefited greatly from medical progress. The emphasis from treatment to prevention of illnesses began to shift dramatically in the late twentieth century. The 1970s ushered in the exercise craze with joggers and runners becoming a commonplace sight along the highways, paths, and sidewalks of every neighborhood. Vitamins and minerals became extremely popular as dietary supplements. In the 1980s, antioxidants (which we just discussed) became the rage. It was as if the whole world of prevention had been born anew. Everyone was talking about antioxidants. Antioxidants were the panacea for prevention. Take your vitamins and live healthier and longer. The 1990s ushered in the decade of herbal remedies and supplements with the same fervor of earlier prevention attempts. Each era of preventive efforts has introduced a new and important aspect toward a better "solution." What about now? What is the new and improved paradigm for prevention of illnesses? In one word, *inflammation*.

Inflammation, or better yet, *inflammation control*, is holding the center stage these days in the world of illness prevention. Inflammation encompasses all of the previous efforts and fads, explaining why and how exercise, antioxidants, and herbs are all effective components to a comprehensive prevention strategy for you. They are part of the solution—but there is more and more evidence that inflammation is at the root of many if not most of our chronic illnesses. As we covered in the previous chapter, *controlling inflammation in your body then becomes the most important single activity you can perform to stay healthy and live a longer, more productive life.* Balance once again enters the picture. Inflammation has been implicated as causally related to the following illnesses or unwanted conditions, most of which are too familiar to Western culture:

- Aging
- Allergies
- Alzheimer's disease
- Arthritis
- Asthma
- Autoimmune diseases such as lupus and AIDS
- Cancer
- Depression
- Diabetes
- Heart disease
- Insomnia
- Obesity
- The metabolic syndrome
- Stroke
- Ulcers

There are many others. Current research on the effects of inflammation on illness development and prevention is some of the most promising ever conducted. You need to know this information. When you understand the implications of controlling inflammation in your body, you will be as astounded and excited as we were in learning of these findings. Inflammation control has become our passion—and it should be yours too.

Homeostasis is vitally involved in the process of inflammation. Your body has to have pro-inflammatory and anti-inflammatory processes to survive. You must have a balance. (Where have you heard that before?) Inflammation is needed to mediate healing. If you have a cut, inflammation fosters the healing process by mustering out the white blood cells and other mechanisms needed to protect the body from foreign invaders (such as bacteria, fungi, and viruses) and to close up the wound. Once healing has been successfully completed, anti-inflammatory processes end the inflammatory attack by white cells and effectively neutralize the attack. "Enough is enough already" was a popular saying in the 1950s, and it applies here.

Unfortunately, the American diet is not balanced. Omega-6, an essential fatty acid found in many vegetable oils and many other food sources, fosters inflammation. Another essential fatty acid, omega-3 (present in many ocean-caught fish, olive oil, and other foods), fosters inhibitory mechanisms that fight inflammation. We have enough pro-inflammatory food in our daily intake to make the ratio of omega-6 to omega-3 an estimated ten to one or even twenty to one in much of the Western world. A ratio of two to one or one to one is considered optimal! That word *balance* pops up again.

Pro-inflammatory processes within the body create chronic irritation of membranes and organs by white blood cells and others. The "bad" cholesterol (LDL) is inflammatory and attaches to vessels to prevent leaks. Too much LDL and chronic, low-level inflammation result in the development of plaque in the vessel and subsequent hardening (athero-sclerosis) and narrowing (occlusion) of the vessels. The "good" cholesterol (HDL) functions to carry the "bad" cholesterol away from the vessel and allows for smooth, unobstructed blood flow. However, if there is too much HDL, vessels can leak and life-threatening hemorrhages may result. *Ad nauseum*, balance and equilibrium are the order of the day for healthy functioning and optimal health. Of course, our diets, being heavily laden with inflammation-fostering substances, result in chronic, low-level inflammation. This imbalance is related to the development of chronic illnesses.

Phytonutrients

Phytonutrients are compounds found in plants (both fruits and vege-tables) that are vital to the long-term health and survival of humans. These chemicals are produced in the plant to protect it from predators such as bacteria, fungi, and viruses. They work in a similar fashion to protect you from free radicals when you ingest them. As opposed to vitamins and other essential nutrients, an absence of phytonutrients in your diet will not result in an immediate or short-term health problem.

They are important, however, in the long-term maintenance of optimal health and longevity. There are literally thousands of phytonutrients in fruits and vegetables. Brightly colored fruits produce phytonutrients, which are anti-inflammatory and have been associated with the prevention of cancer, heart disease, and other chronic illnesses. The deeper the colors of the fruit, the more protective phytonutrients are contained in the fruit.

Which phytonutrients prevent what diseases? How large a "dose" of a particular phytonutrient is needed to prevent a given disease? No one really knows. A single tomato contains hundreds of phytonutrients. Tomato-based foods such as spaghetti sauces seem especially protective against prostate cancer, although no one knows exactly which chemical in the tomato deserves credit. Lycopene currently is receiving most of the credit, but we still don't know for sure. So, what are we to do? We don't know exactly which fruits and vegetables to eat, and we do not know how much. Variety seems to be the rational way to proceed. Using a large number of fruits and vegetables has been shown to render health benefits.

Perhaps it doesn't take a huge amount of a given fruit to render positive health benefits (i.e., anti-inflammatory and antioxidants) but merely a large variety of them. Loading up your diet with a single fruit doesn't make much sense. Loading up your diet with a plethora of fruits does make sense and provides the body with a number of phytonutrients to maintain health and longevity.

In Summary

After a half-century of research, we can still assert that balance is the best way to maintain homeostasis in our bodies: balance in our exercise, diet, and stress management. Fruits serve to complement a healthy lifestyle. They are not drugs or cures for illness. We cannot claim that they prevent or cure any malady. They are natural products that help supply and restore the body to its optimum state, homeostasis. The phytonutrients they contain work synergistically and in harmony with the body to bring it into balance.

Don't expect sudden and stunning results simply by increasing fruits in your diet. You will see small, unnoticed changes in your health with restorative, cumulative benefits over a long period of time. Managing your health is only the beginning of moving from a treatment mentality to a mind-set of being proactive and preventing illness before it occurs.

The Paradigm Shift From
Treatment *to* Prevention

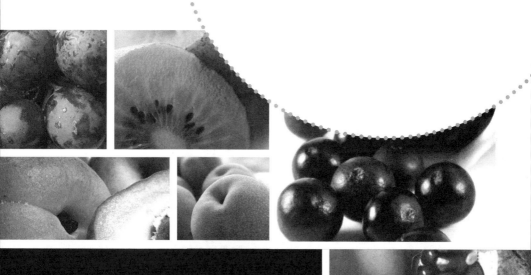

[CHAPTER 4]

DIETARY SECRETS
of the PAST

SOME PEOPLE VIEW THE PALEOLITHIC ERA, THE STONE AGE, WITH a great deal of romanticism. (By the way, *paleo* means "ancient" and *lith* means "stone," so named because of their development and use of stone tools and weapons.) Some scientists believe that these hunter-gatherers lived from (more or less, for you compulsive readers) ten thousand to five hundred thousand years ago. In an idealistic way, we imagine that these people coasted through life happier and healthier than modern-day folks with more leisure time, fewer inequities of class, and free from the many stressors of modern urban life—no traffic to dodge, no bills, and an absence of the fast-food diet. There are those who believe that if we just ate a caveman diet, most of our chronic health problems would disappear. In actuality, the diet consisted of very few simple carbohydrates since agriculture to produce grains had not been developed, and, of course, there were no processed foods. Their diet included meat from wild (and we do mean *wild*) game, fish, some wild fruits, nuts, and tubers with scant amounts of vegetables, vegetable oils, and salts. Unfortunately, the life span of these humans was short, and few lived long enough for us to know whether they would have developed any of the degenerative diseases that afflict today's human beings. So much for romanticism.

Based on what are believed to be 160,000-year-old fossilized human skulls found in Africa, some scientists and paleontologists suggest that these humans were ancestors to modern human beings.[1]

In Creationism, modern-day people are descendants of Adam and Eve, who once lived in the Garden of Eden. In the garden, they could have anything they wanted, except for the forbidden fruit from the tree of the knowledge of good and evil. They were most likely vegans, not killing and eating the animals that roamed paradise with them, but eating "every seed-bearing plant...and every tree that has fruit with seed in it" (Genesis 1:39). The Creation diet probably consisted of wild fruits, vegetables, nuts, and the like. (You can read the description of Creation in Genesis 1–2.)

The introduction of blue-green algae on the world scene years ago began polluting the atmosphere by altering oxygen into free radicals, creating very unstable forms of oxygen. Plants, as a defense mechanism, began to develop antioxidants against these free radicals. The pigment (color) of the plants contained the antioxidants the plants needed to survive by protecting the plants from the very oxygen they produced. Insects rely on the color of plants to find just the right food source for their own antioxidant supply. Animals consumed these plants and commandeered their antioxidant qualities. Much later, humans (like Adam and Eve) began to depend upon fruits, vegetables, and nuts to provide antioxidants, those defenses vital for our long-term survival. Nutritional experts now tell us that the beautiful array of colors in fruits and vegetables represents a variety of antioxidants, not just an attractive harvest cornucopia centerpiece for the Thanksgiving table.

We Are What We Ate

No, that is not a misprint or editorial error. We *are* what we ate.

What happened that made our ancestors dominate the course of history? Success was a function of adaptability. We humans have unique characteristics: our ability to think rationally and logically, to restructure our environment, and to plan ahead. This unquestioned advantage over other species was a result of the frontal cortex of the brain where thinking and reasoning take place. The more advanced our ability to think rationally and logically via an increasing frontal (or neo-) cortex area, the more adaptive we become to an ever-changing environment.

Some scientists believe the diet of these ancient Africans once on the road to oblivion produced modern man. They originally lived in the savanna, a grassy plain with very little forest cover or water. They found their way to the East African Rift Valley and, while scavenging for food, found shellfish along the shores of lakes. These shellfish consumed algae, those simple single-celled organisms we studied in high school biology, and accumulated algae-derived fats in high concentrations, much higher than would have been available on the savanna. These fats were the omega-3s you hear so much about today. They abound in microscopic forms of plant life like the algae. In higher plants, they can be found in leaves, but in lower concentrations. The animals in the Rift Valley ate the algae and the Africans ate the animals, so-called *flesh food*. In this way, the brains of these progenitors of modern man grew and grew, particularly in the frontal cortex, and modern man and woman were born! How fascinating that those two simple substances, water and algae, can account for the progress of human beings.

Some scientists believe that at one point, algae were the only living organisms on the planet. They were made up of a single membrane composed of fat. The ability of nutrients to pass through the membrane was essential to the survival of the algae. Fish and other marine life fed on the algae and produced omega-3 fatty acids. This fish oil was the single most critical dietary component that allowed our ancestors to develop the brain power needed to survive and flourish.*

Even today, we need our brains, but it's to compensate for the disadvantages of modern life. While the Stone Age people had to use their brains to find food to survive, we need to use ours to refuse delicious, tasty, but sometimes harmful foods and to resist the ancient instincts that cry out for us to eat, eat, eat. The Stone Age people used their ingenuity to *save* energy. We may have to find ways to *spend* energy in order to maintain appropriate weight and keep our heart and other muscles fit.

---

* For further information, read *Omega Zone Rx* by Dr Barry Sears (Harper, 2004).

Early men and women, as estimated by nutritionists, consumed about 3,000 calories a day and never gained weight. We consume as little as 2,000 calories a day and have rampant obesity, probably partly because of the nature of our diets and our relative lack of exercise. Unlike our ancestors, we can learn what our bodies need and how they work. We have the advantage.

Appetite and Taste

Our sense of taste is the frontline defense against poisons. People will not eat food that does not taste "right." The second line of defense is the stomach's rejection response. The body vomits or washes out with diarrhea whatever upsets the digestive system. The third line of defense is the liver's filtering and detoxifying system. Liver cells remove the toxins that make their way into the blood supply, rendering those toxins harmless and storing them or releasing them for excretion in the urine. For example, protection against that ancient and familiar substance alcohol is built into the body's genetic code. Alcohol dehydrogenase converts the alcohol into substances such as acetaldehyde, which the body can use or excrete. As long as the liver is not overwhelmed by alcohol, the system works efficiently and effectively.

There are some poisons in which this is not true. Alcohol has been around awhile, and the body has a system for detoxification. However, most additives intentionally put into food, not to mention the pollutants and toxins that accidentally find their way into the food chain, are new to the body, and there is no natural liver enzyme available for defense. If the liver cannot excrete these odd, unfamiliar substances, they can interfere with normal metabolism and cause cancer or birth defects, to mention only two adverse outcomes. But the frontline defense against poisoning is and will remain taste.

Until the end of the Middle Ages, food was not always available. Times of plenty were usually followed by times of famine. The human body adapted to this cycle well, and we became omnivorous, capable of digesting nutrients from both plants and animals. We even have a special enzyme, trehalase, which specifically aids in the digestion of a carbohydrate trehalose, which is unique to the insect exoskeleton. That means we ate insects. We are designed to eat a wide variety of foods and thus survived possible starvation when one or more of our food chain ingredients were in short supply. Moreover, the individual could ingest extra food and the body could store excess energy in its fat tissue when food was plentiful and then call upon these stores when illness or famine occurred.

Today we live in a food-abundant society. The only time we experience famine is during a weight-loss diet. Unfortunately, overeating in susceptible persons may result in diabetes and aggravate high blood pressure, increase the chances of some cancers and intensify arthritis, among other maladies.

Taste and Sugar

Taste perception helps us to avoid harmful plants, signaling that the plant could possibly contain dangerous toxins. The more we're able to discern the bitter taste, the better we can avoid potentially harmful plants. Our taste buds for bitter are in a prominent location, the front of the tongue, for a reason. Some even rest on the lips.

If you have small children, then you know little ones put everything into their mouths. They will rapidly spit out bitter-tasting substances with no prior experience of *sour*. The elderly, after a reduction in their senses and judgment, often revert to the same behavior. This was probably useful to some aging Stone Age folks who may have forgotten or could not see which plants were edible. Bitter meant, "Don't eat this!" During the middle-age years when they were experienced in the safe and not-so-safe foods, they could and often would tolerate bitter foods.

On the other hand, humans who could readily detect sweetness were most likely to survive. Herbivorous (plant-eating) animals will often lick something before eating. Sweet is eaten, sour rejected. Present-day monkeys who actively seek out fruits and berries have larger brains than those who eat leaves of plants close at hand. The hunter-gatherers relished honey and other sources of concentrated sugar such as maple syrup, dried fruit, and honey ants. Starches, the other source of carbohydrate energy, played a relatively minor role in human diets until the start of crop cultivation, including wheat and corn.

So, why do we need sugar? Sugar becomes glucose in our bodies. The brain needs a continual supply of glucose. Glucose is constantly extracted from our blood sugar. Glucose fuels the brain. Sugar is virtually instant energy, providing glucose to feed the brain and power muscle.

The appreciation for the sweet sensation runs deep in the human psyche. It is all over literature and mythology. It has been associated with love and affection in words and phrases such as *sweetie pie, sweetheart,* and *honeymoon.* Our first food, mother's milk, is sweet. Infants smile when given something sweet and cry when given something bitter. This attraction to sweet is not learned, but we are born with it. It is probably related to our brain's need for sugar to manufacture glucose to fuel our brain.

Most of our ancestors had to keep their blood sugar from falling too low since sugar was in short supply. The body uses insulin to metabolize sugar. Insulin is released in our bodies when blood sugar becomes elevated to store the energy in the sugar. It does lower blood sugar, but its main function is to store the energy from sugar for times of future need. When the insulin level is kept low through diet or genetic manipulation, animals live much longer and the rate of aging is reduced dramatically. Low insulin is apparently a signal to the body that energy is scarce. When this happens in animals, they know they need to focus their energy needs on maintaining and repairing themselves so they can outlive the coming famine. An abundance of insulin circulating in our systems from too much sugar results in rapid aging and the major illnesses of aging—diabetes, heart disease, obesity, osteoporosis, dementia, and even cancer. One further point must be noted: our early ancestors had very little sugar available, so those who had "insulin resistance" kept the sugar in the system longer, which fed the brain more glucose (which was in short supply). However, if there is too much sugar in our diets, as is common in most of the Western world, insulin resistance works against us, resulting in obesity and subsequently diabetes.

Sugar enters the body through the digestive system. Sucrose, the sugar found in homes and restaurants around the world, enters the bloodstream as glucose and fructose and then passes through the liver. The entry of glucose into the blood nourishes the brain for about fifteen minutes. Moreover, the presence of glucose causes the pancreas to release insulin, which then stores the glucose in the body's cells. Fructose, in the meantime, is being metabolized in the liver and becomes glucose in about fifteen minutes, which raises the level of blood sugar and again brings out the insulin to store the glucose. This process lasts about fifteen minutes, more or less. So far, the brain has been treated to about thirty minutes of energy in the form of glucose. Finally, if the sugar was eaten in the form of fruit, such as an apple, the fiber in the fruit has trapped the sugar molecules in its weave and releases more sugar molecules in the gut about forty-five minutes after ingestion, giving another thirty minutes of food (glucose) to the brain. Such a process is ideal for the brain's refueling process and defines what we call a *complex carbohydrate*. The process of sugar metabolism is complex, not the carbohydrate. Without the fiber, the sugar's effect is only about fifteen to thirty minutes and defines a *simple carbohydrate*.

The Dangers of High-Fructose Corn Syrup

Japanese researchers invented high-fructose corn syrup (HFCS) as a cheap soft-drink sweetener that has been called by some nutritionists "an unmitigated catastrophe." HFCS is six times sweeter than sucrose and used to sweeten soft drinks, breads, cereals, yogurt, ketchup, and many more commercial products. HFCS is probably safe in moderation, but there are realistic concerns that consumption of a large amount of HFCS causes problems with our lipids, particularly triglycerides (TG), leading to heart problems. In addition, our liver does not handle large amounts of fructose effectively. Liver dysfunction can occur as a result of overuse of fructose. Although one can maintain life with intravenous glucose, IV fructose does not work. Finally, fructose is not well absorbed in the gut and may be a food source for intestinal bacteria with accompanying diarrhea, bloating, and intestinal pain and discomfort. Therefore, it is wise to *reduce dramatically* your intake of HFCS. Of course, the natural fructose found in fruits is present in much lower concentrations and is also accompanied by health-enhancing fiber, minerals, vitamins, and phytonutrients.

Honey was for many centuries the most important source of concentrated sugar, probably rivaling our current use of refined sugar. During medieval times, honey was sold by the gallon or barrel. The wealthy coveted their honey supply. Sweets were in vogue and have remained there without interruption. Not surprisingly, sugar was one of the first crops cultivated deliberately. Sugar cane was first grown in New Guinea and finally in Europe. Both sugar cane and sugar beets have a high concentration of sugar (about 16 percent) and have been commercially produced and sold since about 1600. In the eighteenth century, sugar surpassed honey as the main source of sweetness in Europe. Since the turn of the twentieth century, sugar consumption in the Western world has remained constant, although corn syrup solids and HFCS have partially replaced refined sugars in manufactured products.

Sugar and Its Downside

Sugar is crucial for the care and feeding of the brain. However, it does have significant problems if used in excess. Clearly, there is ample evidence that eating too much sugar can result in obesity. In those populations wherein sugar intake increases, there is a concomitant rise in fat and total caloric intake. At the same time, physical activity decreases.[2] This increase in obesity is attributed to the overconsumption of high-glycemic, simple carbohydrates. There is evidence that eating a meal high in simple carbohydrates results in excessive food intake. It is now believed that body fatness is more related to type 2 (adult onset) diabetes than diet.

When researchers fed rats a diet with sucrose as the only carbohydrate source (a simple carbohydrate), the rats were found to have microscopic damage to the arteries and their blood yielded high amounts of triglyceride and "bad" cholesterol, both implicated in heart disease. Other rats fed simple starches instead of sugar showed no such damage or blood lipid problems.[3] This is similar to what happens in humans when they eat diets high in sucrose and fructose.

A Lesson From the Pima Indians

How does the understanding of the ancients help us in understanding the obesity epidemic and poor health habits of today? The Pima Indians are an excellent modern-day example of the effects of modern lifestyles on our health: "One-half of adult Pima Indians have diabetes, and 95 percent of those with diabetes are overweight."[4] Peter Bennett, a leading epidemiologist, discovered remnants of the Pimas in Sierra Madre, Mexico. The Mexican Pimas were not obese, nor did they share the health problems of diabetes and other degenerative diseases with their Arizona counterparts. The problems of the Arizona Pimas lie in their genes and diet. In their early history before the European migration, Pimas had to possess "thrifty" genes, meaning that their bodies had to store adequate fat in times of plenty to survive famines and droughts. Their hunter-gatherer diet consisted of cholla cactus buds, honey mesquite, poverty weed, prickly pears, mule dear, white-winged dove, jackrabbit, and squaw fish along with cultivated wheat, squash, and beans.

By the end of World War II, the Arizona Pimas had become acculturated into the Western lifestyle; their Mexican brothers continued to eat mostly beans, potatoes, corn tortillas, and an occasional animal product. Pre-agriculture men and women ate lots of protein and fat, so their bodies ideally were insulin resistant, which would minimize the use of glucose, giving them a survival advantage. Since they did not get enough sugar in their diets, glucose was to be saved for brain function. However, a modern diet in highly refined, high-glycemic index carbohydrates has resulted in obesity, diabetes, and cardiovascular disease in the Arizona Pimas. Anthropologists estimated that Mexican Pimas worked an average of twenty-three to twenty-six hours per week while their Arizona cousins worked five hours weekly or less.

The message taken from the Pimas is important. Most of our ancestors survived because they had a genetic predisposition to store fat in times of famine. This predisposition was very useful in surviving the ravages and uncertainties of food availability in the ancient world. Today the overabundance of food, an overconsumption of simple carbohydrates, and a low level of physical exercise are in part responsible for our current obesity and health problems.

Grains

Many health experts extol the virtues of grains as the quintessential source of food on the planet. Not surprisingly, grains became a staple of the human diet when people began to cultivate crops at the dawn of agricultural activities. According to research findings, the frozen, mummified body of Otzi, estimated to be over five thousand years old, was found in the Tyrolean Alps in 1991. His stomach contained grains and meat, suggesting those were the contents of his last two meals.[5]

Grains have vitamins and minerals within, but we humans are not yet biologically capable of taking full advantage of them. Our bodies have not yet adapted physiologically to grains, leaving our guts to inadequately digest and metabolize them. Grains in abundance may actually lead to health problems due to so-called "anti-nutrients," speculated to induce in some people allergen-based disorders and an enlarged pancreas, among other disorders that may occur. From a biological perspective, we are still hunter-gatherers since over 99.99 percent of our genes were developed before the advent of agriculture. Moderation is the name of the game.

When white flour was introduced in the last third of the nineteenth century, it was only available to the rich. Before the invention of roller mills, manual labor was required because the flour had to be sifted by hand through silk filters, over and over, to rid the white flour of the wheat bran and wheat germ. The bran and germ were then fed to the pigs and other farm denizens. The white flour is a simple starch and has a higher glycemic index than sugar. Once ingested, white flour causes a human's blood sugar level to rapidly increase and decrease. A low glycemic index refers to food in which the blood sugar slowly increases and slowly drops. High-glycemic diets are associated with obesity and many diseases, including heart disease, cancer, and diabetes.

Inflammation and Diet

As we mentioned earlier, inflammation is now thought to be at the genesis of many of our chronic diseases. Many of our ancestors followed an anti-inflammatory diet that counteracted our pro-inflammatory genetic proclivities. Thousands of years ago, our diet was rich in fruits, vegetables, lean protein, and omega-3 fatty acids from fish. We ate very little foods containing omega-6, a pro-inflammatory fatty acid. There were no grains or starches. As a result, our inflammatory system was balanced and inflammation was kept at an optimal level. As long as our diets can keep in check our strong insulin and inflammatory responses, then good health is more likely. When this fails to happen, chronic illness is the inevitable result.

About fifty or so years ago, rates of diagnosed heart attacks began to rise. Two factors probably account for this phenomenon. First, infectious diseases and cases of malnutrition began to fall, and people began to live longer. Second, and more importantly, death certificates had new requirements that forced physicians to state the cause of death. "Heart attack" was the easiest and most simple solution to the problem, rather than performing an autopsy. Now, the National Center for Heath Statistics (NCHS) has come to this surprising conclusion: "There is absolutely no evidence that there was an epidemic of heart disease in the 1950s."[6] There have been many fads and myths promulgated by public health officials over the past fifty years with equal lack of data. But who really knows?

Conclusion

Whether you follow the Paleolithic diet or the Mediterranean diet, the ultimate goal is that you include a variety of fruits and vegetables in *your daily diet*. Diets high in sugar, refined carbohydrates, and saturated fats are detrimental to your health, but by now you should know that. In the following chapter, we will examine some new and wonderful discoveries about the power of fruit and fruit juices to your health.

Chapter 5

NEW DISCOVERIES ABOUT FRUIT *and* YOUR HEALTH

T HERE HAS BEEN AN EXPLOSION OF RESEARCH SUGGESTING THAT consumption of fruits and fruit juice is important to remaining healthy. We will not try to look at all the recent articles on fruits and fruit juices and their effects on health, but we will instead give you a sampling of studies of particular interest with regard to several major areas of health. There are many more studies, and the data are piling up! Here are just a few of the findings.

STUDY #1: Alzheimer's Disease

Alzheimer's disease affects millions of people around the world. It is a *neurodegenerative* disease with no clearly defined cause. Like other dementias, it consists of cognitive (memory) decline with sufferers having increasing problems with memory and activities in living.

Alzheimer's consists of brain *plaques* and *neurofibrillary* tangles that accompany the deterioration in functioning. These plaques have been associated with chronic inflammation of the neurons through the substance *beta-amyloid*.

An Alzheimer's patient eventually becomes totally dependent upon caregivers, being completely unable to accomplish even the simplest tasks. In short, it is a progressive, devastating malady. Anything that can help prevent Alzheimer's would be of major benefit to many people.

Could the "Mediterranean Diet" Be Helpful?

The common Mediterranean diet consists of:[1]

- High consumption of fruits, vegetables, breads, beans, nuts, and seeds

- Olive oil

- Dairy products, fish, and poultry consumed in low to moderate amounts; red meat rarely consumed

- Eggs consumed in low amounts

- Wine consumed in low to moderate amounts

By now, you've probably heard of the Mediterranean diet, which consists of a high intake of fruits, vegetables, fish, cereals, and poultry, with a low consumption of red meat, dairy products, and other saturated fats. Olive oil is used frequently in cooking.

Research has evaluated the effects of the diet consumed by residents of approximately sixteen countries that border on the Mediterranean Sea (e.g., Italy, Greece). A study was initiated on 194 patients with diagnoses of Alzheimer's disease and 1,790 without evidence of dementia. The subjects were followed an average of a little over eight years.

The results were quite profound. Those individuals who followed the Mediterranean diet very carefully and consistently reduced their risk of developing Alzheimer's disease by up to 68 percent—a huge amount.[2]

STUDY #2: Alzheimer's Disease

This research was an additional study of Alzheimer's disease prevention, this time specifically testing the effectiveness of fruit and vegetable juices. The study included more than eighteen hundred Japanese Americans as subjects who were sixty-five years of age or older, with an average age of almost seventy-two years. They were initially evaluated between 1992 and 1994 and were all free of the disease. The individuals were followed through 2001.

Subjects were divided into three groups:

- The first group consumed less than one fruit and/or vegetable drink weekly, on average.

- The second group consumed one to two such drinks weekly.

- The third group consumed three or more fruit and/or vegetable drinks weekly.

Those study participants who drank the most fruit and/or vegetable juices weekly had very low rates of Alzheimer's disease at the end of the study. *Their rate of this dementia was an astounding 76 percent lower than those individuals who drank fruit and vegetable juices once weekly or less.*[3]

STUDY #3: Metabolic Syndrome

The metabolic syndrome is a relatively new formal diagnosis in medicine. This syndrome has been shown to *predict heart attacks and diabetes in adults*. Essentially, the metabolic syndrome consists of a group of indictors that all group together to make the diagnosis.

- An important risk factor for this syndrome is the presence of *insulin resistance*, in which the usual amount of insulin fails to work, allowing an abundance of glucose in the blood supply.

- High blood pressure (130/85 or greater), high triglycerides (150 or greater), and low HDL (the "good" cholesterol) must be present.

- An android fat distribution (fat primarily in the stomach and lower abdomen) is present, with an enlarged waist (forty inches or greater in men; thirty-five inches or greater in women).

- Often, markers of inflammation, including TNF-alpha, interleukin 6, and the CRP, are elevated, so inflammation is strongly implicated in the development of the metabolic syndrome.

A research program was conducted in 2005 to evaluate the effects of the DASH (Dietary Approaches to Stop Hypertension) diet on the metabolic syndrome. The DASH diet is similar to other healthy diet routines and consists of reduced calorie consumption, *increased intakes of fruits* (four to six daily), vegetables, low-fat dairy products, and whole grains, along with lowered saturated fats, cholesterol, and sodium (e.g., salt).

The study participants were one hundred sixteen men and women who had been diagnosed with the metabolic syndrome and had agreed to participate in the six-month research. Participants were divided into three groups:

- A control group, who consumed their regular diet

- A second group, who were given a low-calorie diet

- The main experimental group, who were given the DASH diet

The DASH diet resulted in increased HDL ("good" cholesterol), lowered triglycerides, lowered blood pressure, lowered fasting blood glucose, and reduced weight. At the end of the study, all of the individuals in the control group (those who consumed a regular diet) were still diagnosed with the metabolic syndrome. Eighty-one percent of the second group (those who consumed a lower-calorie diet only) remained diagnosable. However, only 65 percent of the DASH diet group continued to suffer from the disease.[4]

Again, we see how important it is to eat large amounts of fruits to give our bodies the fuel they need to fight off and recover from illness.

STUDY #4: Strokes and Heart Attacks

Strokes are another disorder causing disability and death.

In a large, long-term study evaluating the DASH diet guidelines as their focus, researchers summarized data from 88,517 women over a twenty-four-year follow-up period. The data included a close analysis of the women's diets.

The study found that those individuals who closely adhered to the DASH guidelines had significantly fewer strokes and fewer heart attacks than those with low adherence.[5]

Again, eating higher amounts of fruits, vegetables, whole grains, nuts, and low-fat dairy products—and lower amounts of red and processed meats, sodium, and sweetened drinks—has the wonderful effect of helping your body operate at optimum capacity, which in turn gives you the best chance of avoiding illness and increasing both the quality and quantity of life.

STUDY #5: Strokes

In a very comprehensive review of eight studies involving 257,551 subjects who were followed an average of about thirteen years, researchers assessed the effects of eating fruits and vegetables on the chances of having a stroke, either an ischemic (blocked artery) or hemorrhagic (ruptured artery). They divided the subjects into three groups:

- Those who ate less than three servings of fruits and vegetables daily

- Those who consumed from three to five servings of fruits and vegetables daily

- Those who ate more than five servings of fruits and vegetables daily

The findings were consistent with other research on strokes and diet. Both groups that consumed three or more fruits and vegetables daily had clear reductions in the rates of strokes, while the group that ate more than five servings daily *did best*—i.e., they had the least chances of having a stroke of all three groups.[6]

STUDY #6: Asthma, Allergy, and Sinusitis

Asthma, allergies, and sinus problems are a constant malady for many children and adults around the world. Inflammation is clearly involved in all three conditions.

In research on six hundred ninety children (aged seven to eighteen years) from Crete, scientists assessed the effects of the Mediterranean diet on these problems.

The children were grouped as to whether they consumed:

- An optimal Mediterranean diet (high intake of fruits, vegetables, nuts, fish, etc.)

- A moderate-quality Mediterranean diet

- A low-quality Mediterranean diet

The more grapes consumed by the children, the lower the chances of wheezing from asthma. The more oranges and kiwi consumed, the lower their chances of sinus difficulties. Those children with high adherence to the Mediterranean diet experienced the lowest rates of allergy and nighttime coughing, with positive but modest lowering of wheezing episodes. Of interest was the increase in asthmatic symptoms, allergies, and sinusitis with the use of margarine, which often contains saturated vegetable and/or animal oil containing omega 6 fatty acids, known to enhance inflammation.[7]

These findings strengthen the body of research showing that you can reduce your risk of developing illnesses that are caused by chronic inflammation through proper diet and lifestyle changes.

STUDY #7: Cancer, Cardiovascular Disease, and Longevity

If you want to live a healthy and active life, researchers from Britain recently completed a huge study with over twenty thousand participants that provides an excellent guideline.

The subjects were free from cancer and heart attack when first evaluated between 1993 and 1997. They were followed until 2006. The average follow-up length was eleven years.

The participants were given one point each for:

- Not smoking

- Being physically active

- Drinking moderate amounts of alcohol (one to fourteen drinks weekly)

- Eating five or more fruits and vegetables daily

Possible scores ranged from zero to four.

The findings were impressive. Astoundingly, those who scored zero were *four times more likely to die* (most died of cardiovascular disease or cancer) than those who scored four. Those individuals with scores of two were twice as likely to have died as those with a score of four. Moreover, those with scores of four lived an average of fourteen more years than those with scores of zero.[8]

How much more evidence do we need that eating more fruits and drinking more fruit juices, when combined with other healthy lifestyle choices, are important for the prevention of illnesses and maintenance of health?

In Summary

Hopefully, this brief look at some of the most recent and interesting research efforts in the area of illness prevention and fruits has made you aware that you can actually do something about your health: it is up to you.

Eat more fruits and drink more fruit juice starting today. The following chapter will explain the probable mechanisms by which fruits work their magic in our bodies.

[CHAPTER 6]

ANTIOXIDANTS =
"ANTI-RUST" *and*
PHYTONUTRIENTS

W HAT IS IT ABOUT FRUITS THAT MAKE THEM SUCH POWERFUL agents of illness prevention? You now know from research literature that controlling inflammation in your body is the most important single activity you can perform to stay healthy and live a longer, more productive life. So, there must be something in fruits that helps control inflammation. In this chapter, we'll take a look at the specific properties that are involved.

Antioxidants

Antioxidants. That's a buzzword you have probably heard a great deal in the media, but what are antioxidants? In order to understand antioxidants, think of them as "anti-rust" agents that help fight "rust" in the body caused by free radicals.

In the 1980s the antioxidant revolution came on the prevention scene, with many research studies aimed at demonstrating the healing power of vitamins and other natural chemicals that are capable of lessening the effects of *free radicals*—the substances in our bodies that cause "biological rust."

Free radicals (or *reactive oxygen species*, a sinister-sounding name for substances that are the possible causes of horrible diseases) cause cell and tissue damage, leading to illnesses and aging.

Antioxidants

- Antioxidants protect our bodies from wearing down. They strengthen our immune systems, muscles, bones, and skin.

- They do this by stabilizing damage to our cells from free radicals, also known as agents of "biological rust." The more antioxidants present in the body, the less damage free radicals can cause.

- Vitamin C and vitamin E have been among the most mentioned and popularized antioxidants. But there are many more.

Fast forward from the 1980s and exciting news about antioxidants to the past decade, when another new and extremely promising area of research exploded into medical journals and health research publications—*inflammation control.*

In chapter 2, we explored this exciting new concept and how you can use this information to improve your health. In the next few chapters we will:

- Discuss free radicals and oxidation and how they create the inflammation that causes illnesses and aging

- Explain the role that phytonutrients play in reducing your risk of developing diseases

- Explore important fruits and their juices and what they contain to prevent and combat maladies of the human body

- Present some important considerations about fruits, fruit juices, and health in general

Free Radicals and Oxidation

The "rust" in our bodies is due to oxidation by the free radicals as they work to get rid of dead or injured cells. You can see an example of oxidation at work on iron, where actual rust is formed by combining iron with oxygen. You also can see it when you leave an apple slice on the counter and the slice turns brown.

Oxidation is constantly occurring in our bodies too. Day in and day out, the process takes place as a normal physiological function. Defective cells die and are destroyed through oxidation while new cells are born.

When the balance of old and new is maintained, all is well. However, when we have too much oxidation (that is, too many free radicals), our bodies become inflamed, and chronic illnesses can develop.

How Free Radicals Create Chronic Inflammation

There are three conditions that allow free radicals to get out of control and create chronic inflammation:

1. Too much oxidation (too many free radicals are created) in the body (e.g., we eat too much red meat or imbibe soft drinks sweetened with high-fructose corn syrup)

2. Not enough antioxidants (e.g., we fail to consume foods containing adequate vitamin C, omega-3 fatty acids, or other antioxidants)

3. Both, which commonly appears to be the case in our current fast-food culture

Fruits and vegetables are a treasure trove of antioxidants. Clearly, those of you who eat large amounts of fruits and vegetables are getting a good supply of vitamins and other antioxidants.

Exhibit A: The Acai Berry

The acai berry, *sui generis*, is literally in a class of its own. It has the highest antioxidant capacity of any fruit or vegetable. Acai berries are harvested in the Amazon rain forest by local peoples, and there are no protections provided by farmers or other humans while the acai palm matures, so this fruit is completely on its own. The USDA has analyzed 278 fruits, vegetables, and nuts for antioxidant capacity using the ORAC scores we will explain in this chapter. *And the acai berry has one of the highest reported scores for any food.*

The Value of Phytonutrients

As we discovered in chapter 3, another valuable resource found within fruits and vegetables is phytonutrients. Brightly colored fruits produce phytonutrients, which are anti-inflammatory and have been associated with the prevention of several chronic illnesses. How can you tell if the fruit you are eating has a high level of phytonutrients? The deeper the color, the more protective phytonutrients are contained in the fruit.

So, exactly what *are* phytonutrients? Put simply, phytonutrients are natural pesticides in plants. They work to protect plants from many traditional enemies, including bacteria, viruses, molds, and fungi. The more a particular plant has to fend for itself against these and other predators, the more potent the phytonutrient array available to fight the invaders.

There is good evidence of this tendency of a plant to increase its phytonutrient complement when subjected to assaults from the outside.[1] So, you would expect to have an increasing amount of phytonutrients present in organically produced fruits and vegetables as opposed to those produced by conventional methods. Why? Because the conventional farmer does more of the work protecting the plant using pesticides. The organic crop is left more to its own devices and defenses.

However, there is increasing belief among nutritionists and others that a third category of fruits and vegetables has even more phytonutrients, that being those plants that are grown in the jungle or woods or other non-farming environments. Wild fruits are now being shown to have incredible power to ward off invader viruses and other predators. Several have much more potent phytonutrient qualities than any farmed products, organic or conventional.[2]

Once a phytonutrient is developed in a plant and is consumed, you get the benefit of that phytochemical in much the same way as the fruit. Some, not all, of these wild fruits seem to be among the very best sources of phytonutrients, which are very important to our long-term survival and health. Whenever possible, include wild fruits and their juices in your diet. Think of fruits as generators and warehouses of phytonutrients.

There are many particular types of phytonutrients, and more and more are being discovered every year. A particular fruit can have many phytonutrients, but there is still much to learn about which phytonutrients prevent what diseases.

From the research we presented earlier, it is clear that the more fruits, fruit juices, and vegetables you consume, the better your chances are to avoid chronic illnesses. Consuming a wide variety of fruits provides the body with phytonutrients that can help reduce your risk of developing disease and maintain good health.

Our recommendation is to start on your road to healthy living today by consuming a wide variety of fruits and fruit juices. Some of you may feel the results of more phytonutrients in your diets in a few days, and others may experience cumulative effects over a longer period of time.

Methods of Preparation to Best Maintain Phytonutrients

You've probably heard that the methods in which you prepare your fruits and vegetables are crucial to preserving the nutrients in them. Do you steam or microwave? Should you buy foods that are freeze-dried or flash-pasteurized? The list goes on. Preserving those nutrients begins with the moment the produce is harvested.

As soon as a fruit is picked from its tree or vine, the level of phytonutrients begins to diminish. Traditional methods of cooling the fruit during transport and routine pasteurization are not very efficient and, if a fruit is to be squeezed into a juice, may destroy some of the phytonutrients.

However, freeze-drying the fruit preserves the phytonutrient qualities, and flash-pasteurization provides for destruction of unwanted germs without destruction of the phytonutrients. Freeze-drying is a process that makes transportation of fruits much easier. In this process, the fruit is first frozen, then placed under high pressure and heated. The ice (frozen water) in the fruit neatly skips the usual melting phase (where it becomes water) and changes into a gas (water vapor). All that is left is the actual fruit itself, including its phytonutrients, without the water, the freeze-dried product. When water is added to the freeze-dried fruit, *voilà*! Fruit juice with most of its phytonutrients appears.

Flash-pasteurization involves rather rapid heating of a fruit (about fifteen to twenty seconds) to a relatively high temperature (about 160 degrees Fahrenheit). Phytonutrients are preserved by the short time of the process and do not evaporate away. Look for fruit juice products in your local health food store, grocery store, or find an online reputable company that produces a healthy fruit blend using this process.

As we said, there are a lot of phytonutrients in fruits. Here's a brief list of some of the more well-known groups along with the fruits in which they are found:

- Anthocyanins—bilberries, blueberries, loganberries

- Carotenoids—apricots, honeydew melons, oranges, pomegranates

- Flavonoids—acai, blackberries, blueberries, cherries, grapes, plums

- Phenolic acids—aronia (chokeberries), blackberries, grapes, strawberries

- Resveratrol—blueberries, cranberries, grapes

- Tartaric acids—apples, apricots, grapes

This isn't an exhaustive list but rather a small sampling to help you become familiar with phytonutrients. If we listed every phytonutrient and the fruits in which they are found, this book would become encyclopedic!

Phytonutrients work in at least five important ways to assist in illness prevention:

1. In an action similar to musical chairs, some phytonutrients, such as proanthocyanidins (found in cranberries), adhere to cell walls in your body (such as the bladder) so there is no room for bacteria or viruses to attach, keeping you from contracting infections.

2. Phytonutrients act as antioxidants. Flavonoids and carotenoids work to neutralize free radicals so these harmful substances are unable to cause cellular damage and initiate chronic illnesses.

3. Some have antibacterial capabilities, actually killing foreign invaders in your body before they have a chance to get a foothold.

4. Some phytonutrients stimulate or suppress enzymes in your body, allowing the enzymes to interfere with unwanted processes or blocking enzymes from initiating an illness in the first place.

5. Phytonutrients can block the replication of DNA (our genetic code) so cells cannot reproduce unchecked. This is extremely helpful in cancer prevention in which cells can

become out-of-control renegades and start to copy themselves over and over again without limits.

The Rainbow of Health

When it comes to your diet, remember this golden rule: the more colorful your food, the more antioxidants you are getting. "Every hue—green, yellow, orange, red, purple, and even white—signifies a different class of nutrients, each of which offers a unique benefit," says the USDA's Ronald Prior, PhD, one of the first researchers to measure the antioxidants in our food. According to *Prevention* magazine, here's a brief listing of the benefits of each food color group:

1. Yellow/Orange

Sweet potatoes, carrots, pumpkin, mango, corn, and melon all contain a variety of carotenoids, which reduce the risk of developing cancer.

2. Green

Vegetables such as spinach and broccoli are high in lutein, which keeps your vision sharp and clear.

3. Blue/Purple

Blueberries and blackberries are chock-full of anthocyanins, which prevent tumors from forming and suppress their growth.

4. Red

Tomatoes and watermelon are loaded with lycopene, which may protect against cancer and heart disease.

The Rainbow of Health (continued)

5. White

Cauliflower offers the same cancer-fighting benefits as broccoli, its cruciferous cousin, and potatoes are a good source of vitamin C. There's also some evidence that the sulfur compounds in garlic and onions may ward off stomach and colon cancers. Other white foods, like poached chicken, seafood, reduced-fat cheeses, eggs, and tofu, provide all-important protein.

For a truly health-boosting eating plan, mix it up. The key is having a variety of colors at every meal. Research indicates that eating various antioxidants together boosts the overall benefits to your health.[3]

In Search of the Highest ORAC Score

Antioxidants and their targets, the free radicals—also known as reactive oxygen species (ROS)—have a great deal of scientific research associated with them. The free radicals roam around our bodies causing inflammation and disease, being associated with many chronic illnesses such as heart disease and cancer, among others. The more free radicals in your body, the higher the chances are that a chronic illness will manifest itself somewhere. Antioxidants are thought to neutralize the free radicals and thus prevent disease. Antioxidants look for free radicals and scavenge them in a *seek-and-destroy mission.*

To understand this mission, let's go back to our high school chemistry class—Chemistry 101. The free radicals are essentially atoms and molecules "hungry" for extra electrons in their outer orbits. If an atom has the same number of protons (particles with a positive charge) and electrons (particles with negative charges), it is relatively stable and does not engage easily in a chemical reaction. If the outer orbit of an atom is lacking an electron, the atom may attempt to fill or empty the orbit or share electrons with another atom, thus creating as much stability in the new molecule as possible. Atoms can take electrons from other atoms, leaving the "victim" atoms, now free radicals in their own right, to go on their own quests for stability by seeking an electron from still another atom. This can cause a crescendo or cascade within a cell, resulting in cell death—*oxidation*.

As we mentioned earlier in this chapter, oxidation occurs every day in the world around you in the form of rust on iron. Rust will weaken and eventually destroy the metal host upon which it forms if unchecked by paint or other treatment. Oxidation in your body works in the same way to destroy cells. What causes this oxidation to occur in the beginning? Many factors cause oxidative stress on your body's cells, including smoke from tobacco or wood fires, high levels of LDL ("bad" cholesterol) in your blood from fried fast foods, a lack of sleep, aging, and chronic hostility, to name but a few of the purveyors of oxidation in the body. By their very nature, *antioxidants* combat oxidation by providing electrons to needy free radicals, thus creating stable molecules and atoms or destroying them. Once a free radical has been destroyed, it is no longer capable of causing cancers, heart attacks, cataracts, and other illnesses. Examples of antioxidants include vitamins A, C, and E. There are many others. Even calorie restriction appears to work as an antioxidant, as does moderate exercise.

The ORAC (oxygen radical absorbance capacity) score is a very popular method of denoting the ability of an antioxidant to neutralize one of the six free radical classes, *the peroxyl radical.* Using the ORAC score with plants (fruits and vegetables) actually compares the plant's antioxidant potential against a constant, known antioxidant, vitamin E. (Actually, the ORAC score is reported in Trolox units, a water-soluble derivative of vitamin E.) The higher the ORAC score, the more effective the plant's or substance's antioxidant capabilities to seek and destroy free radicals. For example, the cranberry on your Thanksgiving table has an ORAC of about 95, wild blueberries have 92.6, and watermelons have 1.4. The Amazonian palm berry (acai) has an impressive 1,027.[4] Sadly, once this technique was perfected, unscrupulous formulators contrived ways to increase the scores by flooding their products with alpha-tocopherol (vitamin E). Never trust a claim of an ORAC score that does not come from reputable researchers and research laboratories who have published in refereed scientific journals. Often, claims of high ORAC scores are made with no documentation, so do not "swallow" such claims without looking at the source.

Understanding the ORAC

One measure of how much antioxidant power is in various foods is the ORAC (oxygen radical absorbance capacity) test. Eating foods that are high in ORAC value can help you reap the greatest antioxidant benefits to your health and may even slow the aging process in your body and brain. The USDA recommends consuming foods that provide you with 3,000–5,000 ORAC points each day.[5]

What has been done to measure the effects of antioxidants on the other five classes of free radicals? These classes of reactive oxygen species include the hydroxyl radical, hydrogen peroxide, superoxide ion, singlet oxygen, and peroxynitrite. We now have measures of their efficacy to neutralize free radicals, such as the HORAC (hydroxy radical absorbance capacity) and the NORAC (peroxynitrite absorbance capacity), among others.

In order to really know a nutrient's ability to neutralize free radicals, you should probably have access to all these measures instead of one lone ORAC. The ORAC score only tells you the firepower against one particular enemy. You need to see how well the nutrient can seek and destroy all your foes, the six free-radical classes.

The ORAC score and others now used are helpful in determination of relative antioxidant capabilities among various fruits, vegetables, and other foods. However, as we have stressed earlier, more antioxidants may not be better. Avoid overdosing on vitamin supplements. With foods, there is probably no danger of overdosing as long as you eat a variety of foods in moderation.

Top Antioxidant Foods
(ORAC units per 100 grams)[6]

Acai (Brunswick)	18,500
Dark chocolate	13,120
Milk chocolate	6,740
Prunes	5,770
Raisins	2,830
Blueberries	2,400
Blackberries	2,036
Kale	1,770
Strawberries	1,540
Spinach	1,260
Raspberries	1,220
Brussels sprouts	980
Plums	949
Alfalfa sprouts	930
Broccoli florets	890
Beets	840
Oranges	750
Red grapes	739
Red bell peppers	710
Cherries	670
Onion	450
Corn	400
Eggplant	390

Some nutritional experts have speculated that the ORAC measures the ability of the antioxidants in food to prevent the formation of free radicals before they start. Assays such as the ORAC and HORAC are not a substitute for scientifically controlled studies that test for the effects of a particular fruit or variety of fruits on the health and longevity of human beings. Although we may someday have a recommended daily intake (RDI) of antioxidants (as measured by the ORAC, NORAC, and the like), we do not have any such RDI today and probably will not see it in the near future.

Balance, Variety, and Moderation

There is no consensus in the scientific community for making antioxidant recommendations. Some studies have suggested that higher doses of supplemental antioxidants may lower the risk of cancer, dementia, and cardiovascular disease, while others have found them to be ineffective or possibly even harmful. This leaves the consumer confused and often at the mercy of those who employ scare tactics to either avoid or endorse the taking of antioxidant supplements based on one-sided philosophies. When it comes to fitness and nutrition, balance, variety, and moderation are the key to antioxidant supplementation.

Many promoters of antioxidants would have us believe that free radicals are responsible for all the ills that plague humanity. Every day our bodies face ten thousand or more attacks from these highly reactive oxygen species that try to stabilize themselves by stealing electrons from other cells. External sources such as UV rays, the ozone layer, drugs, extreme exercise, food additives, stress, radiation, air pollution, high-fat diets, obesity, organic solvents, tobacco smoke, and pesticides also contribute to the vast free-radical pool. When oxidation becomes excessive, there is damage to our cells, which alters their structure and function. The outcome results in over fifty identified medical illnesses (cardiovascular disease, cancer, macular degeneration, and Alzheimer's disease, to name just a few).

"This oxidative stress is damaging in some contexts, but probably beneficial in others," concludes Walter Bortz of Stanford University

School of Medicine. Free radical production occurs every day and every minute of our lives. These unpaired electrons are a natural byproduct of the metabolic process that combines the oxygen we breathe with the food we eat to produce energy. These reactive oxygen species (ROS) are crucial to our immune system to fight off bacteria and viruses that cause infection. They help destroy cancer cells and decrease the production of LDL (the bad cholesterol). Considering all these benefits, the previous view that all oxidative stress is bad is probably an oversimplification.

Antioxidants scavenge and neutralize free radicals. In this way, they can protect against the progressive oxidative damage and the onset of diseases. Recommendations for antioxidant usage are based on more than two hundred studies of antioxidants conducted over the last twenty years. Clinical trials on patients with disease (the response may be different in healthy individuals) show that antioxidants offer potential protection against:[7]

- Macular degeneration, prostate cancer, and respiratory infection: Strong

- Parkinson's and Alzheimer's: Promising

- Diabetes: Suggestive

- Arthritis, heart disease, and lung cancer: Weak

However, there are literally thousands of compounds, produced both by our bodies and from plant sources, that demonstrate this capability. Only certain antioxidants work in certain situations, and all antioxidants may not be the optimal one for that specific body tissue. Like a finely tuned orchestra, they perform best when they are performing together. "We do not understand the intricate relationship between certain types of antioxidants and certain types of free radicals at different moments over the course of one's lifetime."[8]

Problems arise with antioxidants when overzealous individuals consume excessive amounts and buy into the hype of often well-intentioned but misinformed supplement pushers. Bortz says that "antioxidants in high doses may do the body harm.... We simply don't know yet which ones do which and when."[9] High doses tend to disrupt the body's delicately balanced defense system. That is why it is important to adhere carefully to the following recommended daily allowances.

The Importance of Reference Values

Three important types of reference values included in the dietary reference intake (DRI) are recommended dietary allowances (RDA), adequate intakes (AI), and tolerable upper intake levels (UIL).

The RDA recommends the average daily dietary intake level that is sufficient to meet the nutrient requirement of nearly all (97 to 98 percent) healthy individuals in each age and gender group.

An AI is set when there is insufficient scientific data available to establish an RDA (for example, 15 mg or 22.5 IU of vitamin E for men and women). AI meets or exceeds the amount needed to maintain a nutritional state of adequacy in nearly all members of a specific age and gender group.

The UIL is the maximum daily intake unlikely to result in adverse effects. The Institute of Medicine (IOM) reviewed three hundred forty peer-reviewed scientific vitamin E studies and references. They concluded that vitamin E is safe at levels as high as 1,500 IU (international units) per day for natural vitamin E, or 1,000 IU for the synthetic form.[10] There are no changes in platelet aggregation or adhesion with daily vitamin E intakes as high as 1,200 IU.[11] Over twenty years of previous reports show a lack of toxicity in human supplementation of vitamin E.[12] Research reports that more than 10 percent (14 percent among whites) of U.S. adults take doses of 400 IUs or more of vitamin E per day. The CDC's Dr. Earl S. Ford noted, "If people who consume 400 IU or greater of vitamin E per day are indeed at increased risk for premature death, a sizeable percentage of U.S adults fall into this risk group....Furthermore, a report showing that 64 percent of health care professionals had a daily vitamin E intake of 400 IU or greater suggests that [they] may need to reconsider the use of high doses of vitamin E."[13] Even Dr. Andrew Weil, the recognized authority on alternative medicine among mainstream medical practitioners, is quoted as saying even after all the negative press, "I still recommend taking 400 IU of vitamin E in the form of mixed tocopherols and tocotrienols for general antioxidant and protective effects. I would like to see more research assessing the health benefits of the whole natural E complex."[14]

There is considerable rebuttal and criticism of the reports that claim vitamin E supplementation is not effective and may even be harmful. Supporters of supplementation say the negative reports create unnecessary fear. The criticism of high doses of vitamin E are oversimplified and sensationalized because they are designed to sell newspapers and support the pharmaceutical industry. The form of vitamin E should be the d-, or natural, form and not the dl-, or synthetic, form. The dl- molecule has a shape that the body is not designed to handle, whereas the d- form is the only configuration the body is able to use.[15] The recommendation is 400 IU of vitamin E (as d-alpha or mixed tocopherols) and 200 mcg of selenium for general antioxidant protection.[16] Its effect on the healthy population needs to be differentiated from trials where patients were in poor health and exposed to high levels of oxidative stress (cancer, heart disease, vascular disease, diabetes, overly medicated, smoking, etc.). Healthy people can derive many long-term benefits from vitamin E, such as a reduction in oxidative cell damage and inflammation.[17] The statistical reviews (meta-analysis) could be skewed, and there appears to be a financial conflict of interest (pharmaceutical companies, CODEX). With all of the negative press that vitamin E has received in recent years, one almost wonders whether there's a government conspiracy behind it all or the CDC isn't just up to speed on the latest research about vitamins.[18] Even if we take their word for it that beta-carotene in the form of supplements has not been proven to protect against cancer, it is still believed that beta-carotene may work in combination with phytonutrients, vitamins, and other naturally occurring food substances.[19]

It is not the purpose of this text to bash the use of antioxidants or to question their importance. Rebuttals criticizing the research both for and against the use of antioxidant supplements abound. There is a delicate balance between free radicals and antioxidants in the body. The antioxidants and other healthful nutrients in food also work in a fine

ACAI BERRY

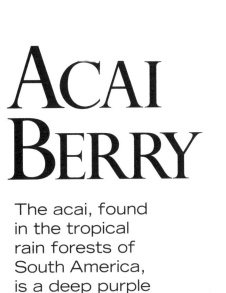

The acai, found in the tropical rain forests of South America, is a deep purple berry, about an inch in diameter.

Of all fruits, vegetables, and nuts known in the world today, none have a higher total ORAC score than acai. The ORAC score of freeze-dried acai is 1,026—more than ten times higher than cranberries.

ACEROLA

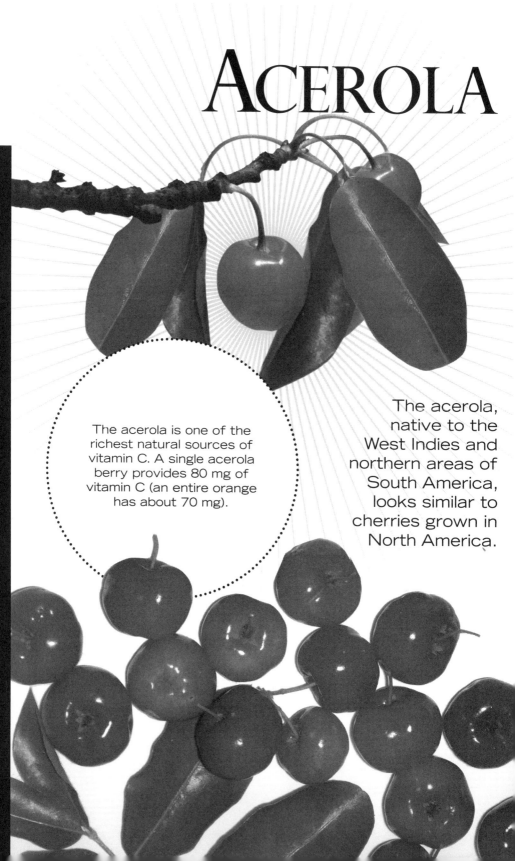

The acerola is one of the richest natural sources of vitamin C. A single acerola berry provides 80 mg of vitamin C (an entire orange has about 70 mg).

The acerola, native to the West Indies and northern areas of South America, looks similar to cherries grown in North America.

APRICOT

Apricots are similar to a small peach, ranging in color from dark yellow to dark orange.

The apricot contains important antioxidants and phytonutrients, as well as a very ample supply of beta-carotene.

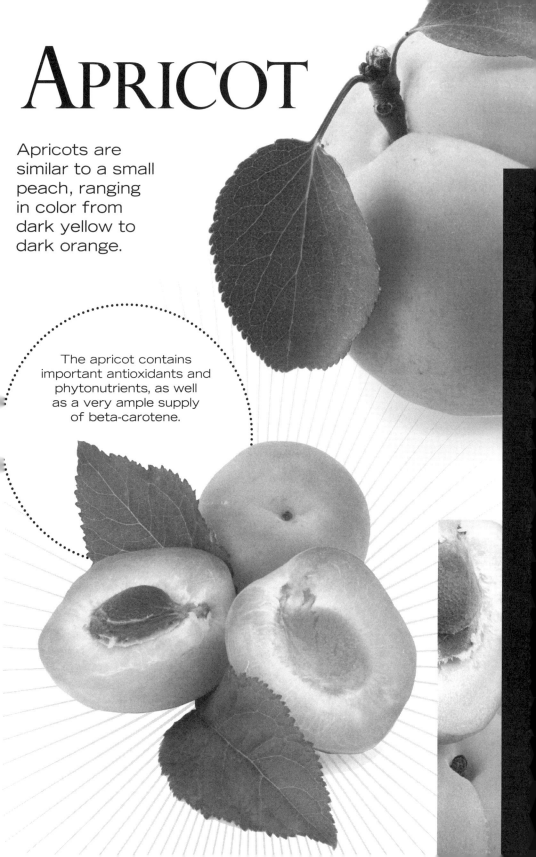

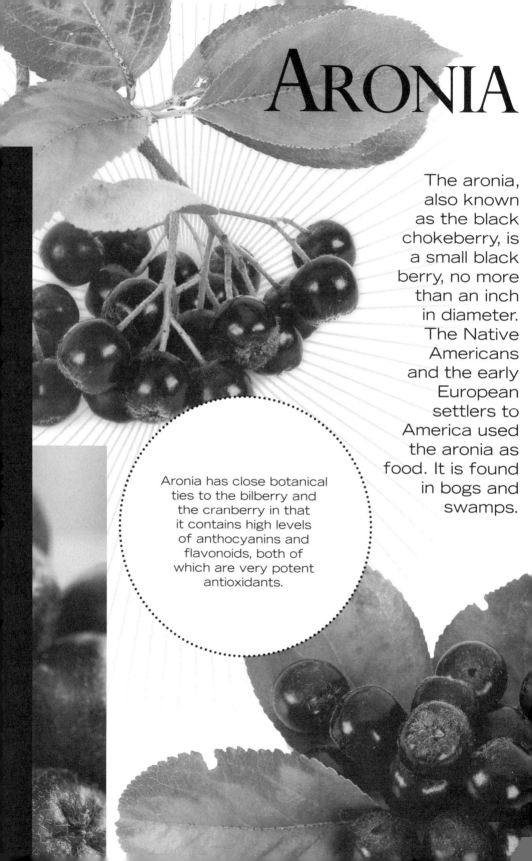

ARONIA

The aronia, also known as the black chokeberry, is a small black berry, no more than an inch in diameter. The Native Americans and the early European settlers to America used the aronia as food. It is found in bogs and swamps.

Aronia has close botanical ties to the bilberry and the cranberry in that it contains high levels of anthocyanins and flavonoids, both of which are very potent antioxidants.

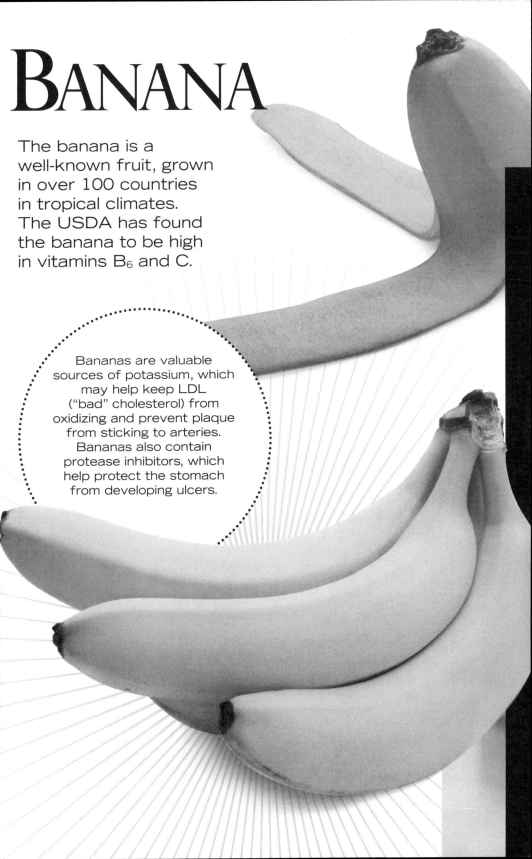

BANANA

The banana is a well-known fruit, grown in over 100 countries in tropical climates. The USDA has found the banana to be high in vitamins B_6 and C.

Bananas are valuable sources of potassium, which may help keep LDL ("bad" cholesterol) from oxidizing and prevent plaque from sticking to arteries. Bananas also contain protease inhibitors, which help protect the stomach from developing ulcers.

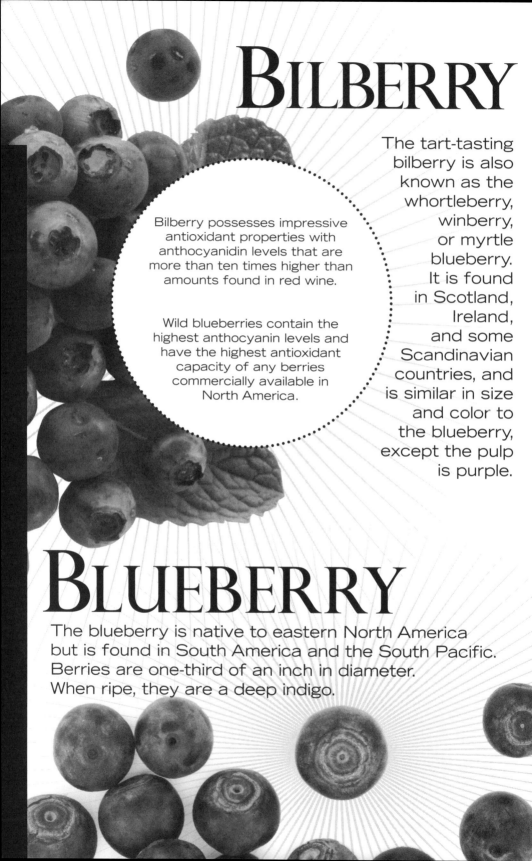

BILBERRY

The tart-tasting bilberry is also known as the whortleberry, winberry, or myrtle blueberry. It is found in Scotland, Ireland, and some Scandinavian countries, and is similar in size and color to the blueberry, except the pulp is purple.

Bilberry possesses impressive antioxidant properties with anthocyanidin levels that are more than ten times higher than amounts found in red wine.

Wild blueberries contain the highest anthocyanin levels and have the highest antioxidant capacity of any berries commercially available in North America.

BLUEBERRY

The blueberry is native to eastern North America but is found in South America and the South Pacific. Berries are one-third of an inch in diameter. When ripe, they are a deep indigo.

CAMU CAMU

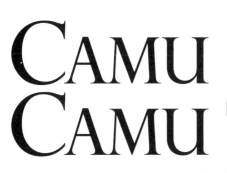

As the world's richest natural source of vitamin C, camu camu is said to contain 30–60 times more vitamin C than an orange. Oranges provide 500–4,000 ppm vitamin C; camu camu provides up to 500,000 ppm.

The camu camu is another gift from the Amazon and looks very similar to a cherry although with a reddish-purple tint.

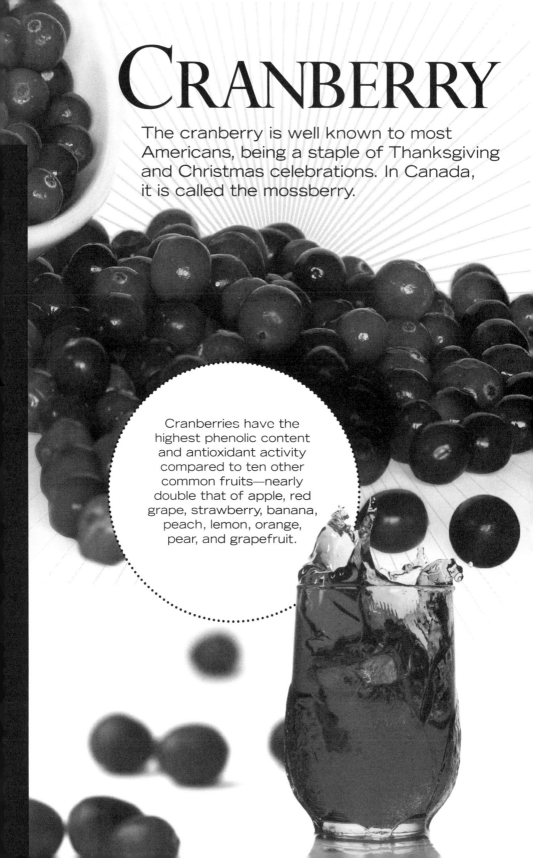

CRANBERRY

The cranberry is well known to most Americans, being a staple of Thanksgiving and Christmas celebrations. In Canada, it is called the mossberry.

Cranberries have the highest phenolic content and antioxidant activity compared to ten other common fruits—nearly double that of apple, red grape, strawberry, banana, peach, lemon, orange, pear, and grapefruit.

Kiwi

The kiwi is native to China
and has been called the
Chinese gooseberry, melonette,
and, most recently, the kiwifruit.
The fruit has a fuzzy skin,
is the size of a large
chicken egg, and
is greenish-brown.

Kiwi skews the nutritional
grading curve. A recent
study at Rutgers University
found kiwifruit, with an
index of 16, to be the most
nutrient dense
of all fruits.

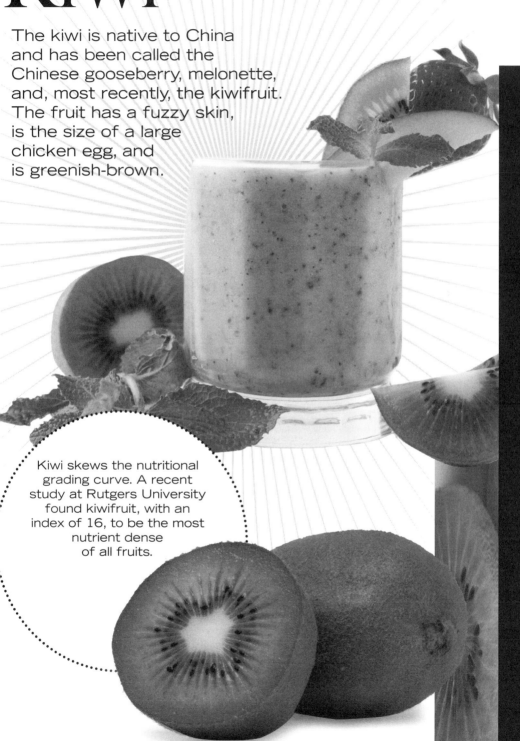

LYCHEE FRUIT

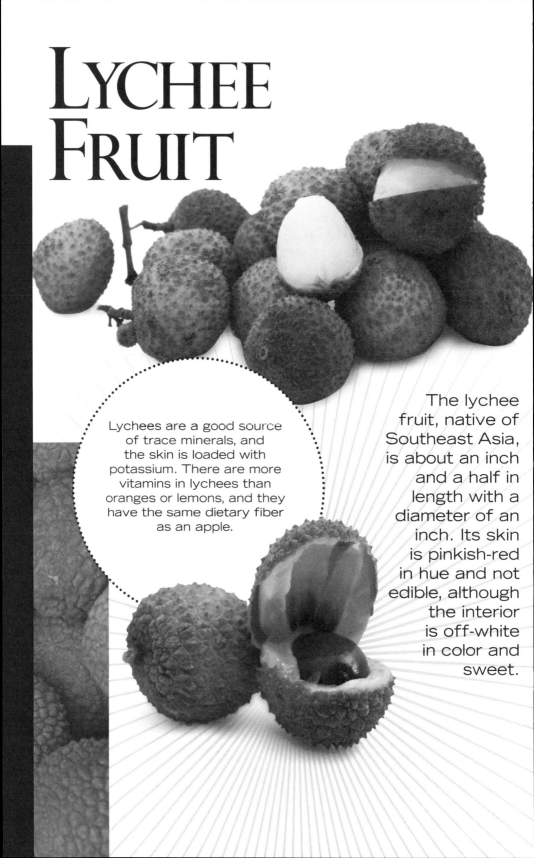

Lychees are a good source of trace minerals, and the skin is loaded with potassium. There are more vitamins in lychees than oranges or lemons, and they have the same dietary fiber as an apple.

The lychee fruit, native of Southeast Asia, is about an inch and a half in length with a diameter of an inch. Its skin is pinkish-red in hue and not edible, although the interior is off-white in color and sweet.

NASHI PEAR

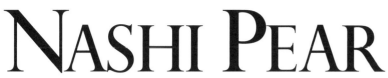

The Nashi pear is named for the area of China where it is natively grown. It has also been called the Asian pear, sand pear, and apple pear. The pear actually is about the size of an apple with round shape.

Nashi pears contain antioxidants, including vitamins C and B-complex. Iodine and phosphorous are also found in the Nashi pear.

Pears contain vitamins C, E, and B_2 as well as phytonutrients.

PEAR

Pears we consume in the United States today are one of the Nashi's offspring. Pear seeds first came to North America via early settlers in Massachusetts. The fruit is usually about four inches tall and two and one-half inches in diameter.

PASSION FRUIT

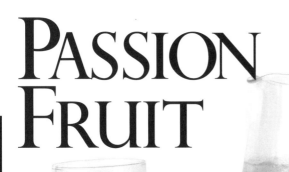

Two passion fruits provide only 34 calories. Eaten with seeds, passion fruits are an excellent source of fiber, with nearly 4 grams in two fruit servings.

Passion fruit was so named by Spanish explorers to South America because the fruit's flower was thought to exhibit several symbols of the crucifixion of Christ. Passion fruit can grow to about the size of a grape-fruit and is yellow in color.

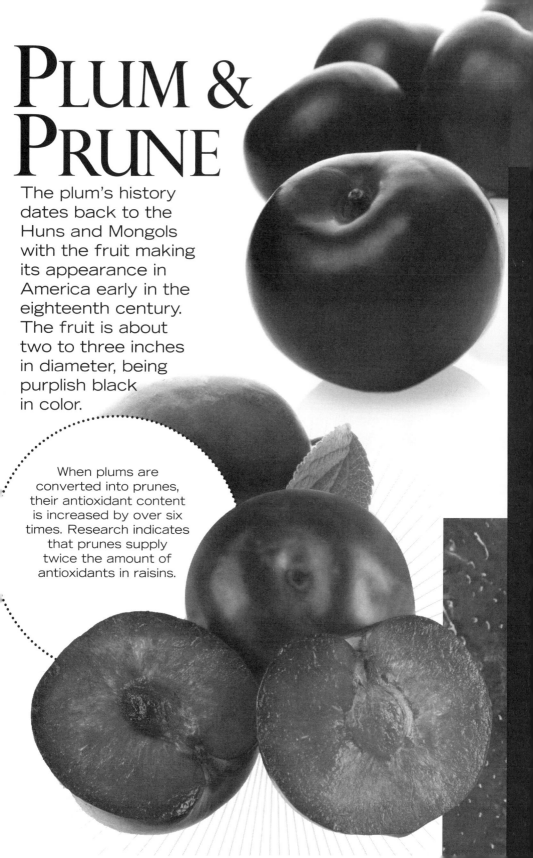

PLUM & PRUNE

The plum's history dates back to the Huns and Mongols with the fruit making its appearance in America early in the eighteenth century. The fruit is about two to three inches in diameter, being purplish black in color.

When plums are converted into prunes, their antioxidant content is increased by over six times. Research indicates that prunes supply twice the amount of antioxidants in raisins.

POMEGRANATE

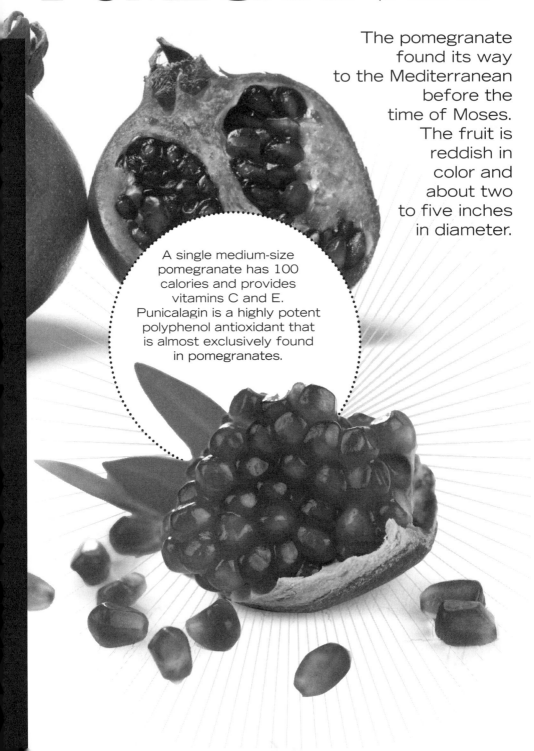

The pomegranate
found its way
to the Mediterranean
before the
time of Moses.
The fruit is
reddish in
color and
about two
to five inches
in diameter.

A single medium-size
pomegranate has 100
calories and provides
vitamins C and E.
Punicalagin is a highly potent
polyphenol antioxidant that
is almost exclusively found
in pomegranates.

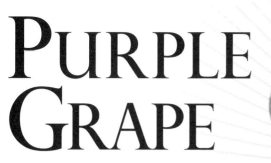

PURPLE GRAPE

The purple grape has been an important component of the diet of the Mediterranean countries for eons, but it made its initial appearance in America in the seventeenth century.

Grape seed offers the highest concentrations of polyphenols in nature. OPC, the most potent free-radical scavenger with an antioxidant effect up to fifty times more potent than vitamin E and up to twenty times greater than vitamin C, is derived from grape seed.

WHITE GRAPE

The white grape is actually not white, but pale green.

WOLFBERRY

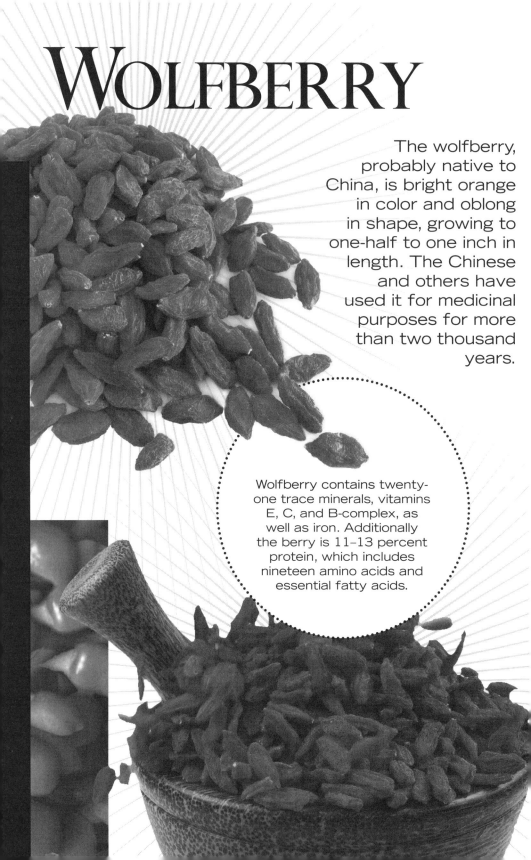

The wolfberry, probably native to China, is bright orange in color and oblong in shape, growing to one-half to one inch in length. The Chinese and others have used it for medicinal purposes for more than two thousand years.

Wolfberry contains twenty-one trace minerals, vitamins E, C, and B-complex, as well as iron. Additionally the berry is 11–13 percent protein, which includes nineteen amino acids and essential fatty acids.

balance, which scientists are just beginning to understand. The takeaway message is that it is best to get most of your antioxidants through foods like fruits and vegetables, where they exist in the proportions nature intended. Antioxidants protect one another from oxidation, and if one is lacking, another can become a pro-oxidant.

We believe you should get nine servings of fruits and vegetables per day. This should include at least three servings of a variety of bright deep-pigmented fruits. It would be naïve to think this is always possible, so if you must supplement, adhere to the concept of moderation. Also, include a source that provides a mixture of all naturally occurring forms of vitamin E—α (alpha), β (beta), δ (delta), and γ (gamma) tocopherols and tocotrienols. The acai berry is an excellent source of the highly beneficial gamma form of vitamin E as well as the other tocopherols.

Science has learned and is currently aggressively reporting that inflammation is the "real" culprit in the disease process. Excessive oxidation may not be the key factor in disease development at all. Inflammation plays the biggest role in "chronic" disease, and free radicals may trigger the inflammatory response. To this end, antioxidants may assist in preventing or help control inflammation. Antioxidant vitamins, and more importantly phytonutrients, have a cumulative role in contributing to minimize or prevent inflammation. How to address chronic "silent inflammation" is the new paradigm in today's health initiative. And just like free radicals, inflammation can also be beneficial. So an overabundance of anti-inflammatory agents is not recommended if the delicate balance is offset. So balance, moderation, and variety once again will play a part in those individuals who will emerge with a better understanding of how to care for their health and live a long and productive life.

In the next chapter, we will outline a few facts about some of the more interesting fruits available and give you basic information about each fruit. We will mention a cross-section of them to acquaint you with the wide variety of fruits you could—and should—be consuming for better health outcomes.

CHAPTER 7

The 411 *on* FRUITS

Y OU MAY HAVE HEARD THE NAMES OF MANY FRUITS BUT KNOW nothing about them or their histories. Perhaps you have never seen a camu camu or a lychee fruit. How about an acerola or an aronia? A Nashi pear or a bilberry?

In this chapter, you will learn about the difference between acid-forming fruits and alkaline-forming fruits. Then we highlight a number of our favorite fruits. Some will have familiar names; some will not. Hopefully, you will want to try some of the new ones and return to consuming some of the more common fruits you may have forgotten.

Remember, no single fruit can possibly meet all the requirements of phytonutrients needed in your diet. *Variety* is the spice of life! It should be one of your two most favorite words (along with fruit): variety—fruit—variety—fruit—variety—fruit.

Tips for Selecting and Storing Fresh Fruit

Follow these tips to ensure you enjoy your fruit at its best.

Fruit	At the Market	At Home
Bananas	Purchase bananas that are slightly green at the tips with as few marks or scratches as possible.	Store bananas on the counter until they are ripe.
Berries (all types)	Purchase berries that are dry and plump; mushy or shriveled berries are overly ripe.	Refrigerate berries, covering the container. Don't wash until ready to serve.
Grapes	Look for bunches with green stems and firm fruit that is still attached to the stem.	Refrigerate grapes. Don't wash until ready to serve.
Kiwi	Purchase fruit that smells fruity and is slightly spongy when squeezed (not too hard and not too mushy).	When storing kiwi, watch for loss of fuzz as this is a sign that the fruit is becoming overripe.
Pears	Purchase pears that are firm, not soft. A soft or mushy pear is on its way to being overly ripe.	Ripen hard pears in a paper bag at room temperature. Store ripened pears in the refrigerator.

Fruit	At the Market	At Home
Peaches, plums, and apricots	Purchase fruit that smells fruity and is slightly spongy when squeezed (not too hard and not too mushy).	If fruit is too hard when you purchase it, soften it in a paper bag at room temperature.

Before we discuss the health benefits of various fruits, let's take a long, hard look at a hot topic on the subject of naturopathic health and nutrition—the pH balance of your diet.

The pH Factor

What implication does pH of products have on your health? Some in the naturopathic field believe that many people are walking around too acidic because of diet, and this is the cause of aging and disease.

"Sounds like a good theory," you might be saying to yourself. Then why is it such a hot topic? Because one author labels a certain food as acidic while another calls it alkaline. "If you collect a number of books, brochures, pamphlets and health guides from a variety of sources, you will find that they contradict each other," says Stephen Cherniske, MSc. "Some devise entire charts based upon invented terminology, such as sub-acid, and acidifying, forgetting that these foods will be swallowed into a stomach that is hundreds of times more acidic than the most acidic food on their list!

"Then there are the blatant contradictions in books that warn sternly against eating acidic foods, but recommend that you take HCl (hydrochloric acid) as a digestive aid or consume apple cider vinegar (acetic and malic acid) for just about any ailment."[1]

So, what is a health-conscious consumer to do? Are these acid/alkaline lists useless? According to Cherniske, the answer is yes. "If you have such a list on your refrigerator and you have been trying to reconcile the contradictions between different health gurus, you can now throw the list away and relax."[2]

Chemistry 101: Acid vs. Alkaline

Have you forgotten the difference between an acid and a base? Here's a quick refresher from your high school chemistry class.

When you mix an acid with water, it turns litmus paper red, tastes sour, and releases hydrogen ions. Depending on an acid's concentration of hydrogen ions, it can be weak or strong, and this strength is measured on a pH scale. Pure water registers as 7.0 on a pH scale, and this is considered the neutral point. The more acidic a substance is, the lower the pH level below 7.0.

When you mix an alkaline (or base) substance with water, it turns litmus paper blue, tastes bitter, and accepts hydrogen ions. Bases are also measured on the pH scale, and the stronger the base, the higher the pH above 7.0.

Cherniske attributes the widespread confusion to the fact that there are four distinct acid/alkaline factors in human health and nutrition, and when authors only focuses on one factor or another, contractions can abound.

Here are the four acid/alkaline factors as described by Cherniske:[3]

1. Acid/alkaline balance

According to Cherniske, acid/alkaline *balance* refers to the pH level of your blood, which must be kept around 7.4. Your body maintains this balance through buffer systems in your blood and pH-regulating action of your lungs and kidneys.

> ### Quick Definitions
>
> *Acidosis* occurs when your blood's pH level dips below 7.35. When this happens, your lungs pick up the pace, making you breathe more rapidly in order to remove carbonic acid as you exhale carbon dioxide (CO_2). Meanwhile, your kidneys increase the acidity of your urine, and balance is quickly restored.
>
> *Alkalosis*, as you probably guessed, is the opposite of acidosis and can occur if you hyperventilate or lose stomach acid due to excessive vomiting or overuse of antacids and/or ulcer medications. When alkalosis occurs, your breathing becomes shallower and your urine more alkaline.

2. Acid/alkaline quality of foods

Cherniske says, "Fruits are sometimes classified as acid, sub-acid, or sweet. This differentiation has nothing to do with the acid/alkaline balance in the blood, which is not affected at all by the acid content of a food.... The only reason to classify fruits this way may be to help in the botanical description of the food. For example, oranges, grapefruit, lemons, limes, tangerines, and kumquats are citrus fruits containing citric acid. Apples, sometimes classified 'sub-acid,' contain malic acid. Cranberries contain benzoic acid."[4]

3. Acid/alkaline chemistry of digestion

In spite of the fact that many advertisements preach the benefits of "neutralizing stomach acid," the hydrochloric acid (HCl) secreted by the cells in the lining of your stomach plays a crucial role in healthy digestion. The normal pH level of your stomach should be somewhere between 1.5 and 2.5 (very acidic). According to Cherniske, "By the time your food has been reduced to a semi-liquid mass called *chyme*, its pH is far less acidic (in the range of 3.5 to 5.0), and it is ready to pass into the small intestine.

"Digestion continues in the small intestine by the action of enzymes secreted by the pancreas, gallbladder, and intestinal wall. But a fundamental difference exists here. Whereas the initial stages of digestion in the stomach required a highly acidic medium, the latter stages require an alkaline environment. This is because over 90 percent of all absorption takes place in the small intestine, and absorptive tissue is extremely sensitive. This rapid and dramatic change in pH to alkaline is accomplished by the pancreas, which secretes the necessary quantity of bicarbonate."[5]

4. Acid/alkaline residue of foods after digestion

According to Cherniske, in the final stages of your body's process to turn food into energy, the mineral content of food leaves a residue in your system that is either alkaline, acid, or neutral, depending on the mineral makeup of that particular food. Sulfur, phosphorus, and iron are found primarily in proteins, such as meat, fish, poultry, eggs, grains, and most nuts. That's why these foods are referred to as acid-forming foods. Soft drinks are an example of a food product that contains no protein but lots of phosphate, and thus is very acid forming. Potassium, calcium, magnesium, and sodium are found primarily in fruits and vegetables, and because they form alkaline reactions in your body, they are called alkaline-forming foods.

Why Balance Matters

By now you're probably thinking, "Thanks for the science lesson, but what does this have to do with my food choices?" It's important to understand these four keys to acid/alkaline balance because you probably consume what is called the "standard American diet" (ironically abbreviated as SAD), which is extremely acid forming. It's no surprise to most people that surveys reveal Americans consume more soft drinks than any other beverage while consumption of alkaline-forming vegetables and fruit is at an all-time low. The result is widespread acidosis, which accelerates catabolic damage and impairs anabolic repair processes.

Does this mean that we should all be taking antacids? Cherniske says no. "Antacids have been shown to seriously reduce nutrient bioavailability. A more sensible conclusion is that we should eat less meat and more fruits and vegetables."[6]

In summary, acid and alkaline foods are neither good nor bad. The pH of a product is not that important to the body's overall pH balance. Many fruits are acidic in nature but tend to leave an alkaline residue in the body. The question should be not is the product acidic, but whether it is acid forming. The pH of fruit juice is acidic in order to maintain an environment that prevents the growth of harmful microorganisms. Overall, juices do not increase the acid load on the body.

Now let's take a look at a variety of fruits that are beneficial to your overall health. We've selected some that we believe to contribute the most in terms of antioxidants and phytonutrients. To help you identify some of the rarer fruits mentioned, you can find photographs of each of these fruits, along with a recap of some of the key facts about them, in the photo section at the beginning of this chapter.

Acai Palm

The acai palm, acai berry or just plain acai (*Euterpe oleracea*), is found in the tropical rain forests of South America.

- It is a deep purple berry, about an inch in diameter.

- The berries grow on palm trees that reach up to 90 feet in height, being quite majestic to behold.

- In the language of locals, *acai* means "the fruit that cries."

- The original inhabitants, according to regional folklore, believed that the acai provided incredible energy to its users, very important for survival in a primitive, hostile environment with enemy warriors a constant threat.

- Brazilians who live in or near the region of the acai eat it regularly and ascribe to it numerous healing qualities, including stopping tooth decay, improving skin diseases, and preventing illnesses in general. The Caboclo consists of three tribes indigenous to the rain forest of Brazil. According to one study, the acai palm accounts for a little more than two-fifths of the Caboclo's diet by weight![7] That is a whole "bunch" of acai.

- Of special importance is the fact that the acai is harvested after having grown wild, which means that the fruit is likely to be loaded with phytonutrients.

No single fruit can do everything. However, in our opinion, the closest nominee to a complete fruit is undoubtedly the acai.

- The acai is rich in antioxidants (vitamin A, calcium, amino acids, and some vitamin C), omega-3 fatty acids, fiber, proteins, carbohydrates, and minerals.

- Of particular interest to disease prevention capability is the variety of phytonutrients in the acai. The acai contains a large number of differing phytonutrients from the families of anthocyanins and flavonoids, including proanthocyanidin and resveratrol.[8]

- Anthocyanins, found in the skin of the acai, are responsible for the red, blue, to dark purple or black color when mature and appear to act as a sunscreen for the fruit. The level of anthocyanins is five times more potent than when found in other fruits.

- Other phytonutrients found in acai include catechin and epicatechin, kaempferol, eriodictyol and erodictyol-7-glucoside, luteolin, luteolin-4-glucoside, chrysoeriol, quercetin-3-arabinoside, and isoquercitin.

- Of all fruits, vegetables, and nuts known in the world today, none have a higher total oxygen radical absorbance capacity (ORAC) than acai. The previous highest ORAC for a food was cranberries, at 92.55. The ORAC score of freeze-dried acai is 1,026—more than ten times higher than cranberries.

Acai has the highest superoxide scavenging activity of any fruit, vegetable, or nut based on the S-ORAC (super-oxygen radical absorbance capacity); both a slow and fast antioxidant based on the total antioxidant (TAO) assay; peroxynitrate radical scavenging activity based on the NORAC assay; and hydroxyl radical scavenging activity based on the HORAC assay.

With its many exciting properties, the acai should be an important and integral part of your anti-inflammatory program. How can you get your hands on some acai? It is not easy, since the distance from the Amazon rain forest to your kitchen is several thousand miles in most cases! Fortunately, the berry is now found in excellent fruit juice blends. Look for a blend that incorporates whole fruit, skin, pulp, and seed; is minimally processed so that the juice contains live and active enzymes; and does not include high-fructose corn syrup (HFCS) or is diluted with added water. Enjoy its benefits!

Acerola

The acerola (*Malpighia glabra*) is also known as the Caribbean cherry, West Indian cherry, Barbados cherry, Surinam cherry, and wild crape myrtle. As a few of its names imply, the acerola is native to the West Indies and northern areas of South America. It looks similar to the wild and sweet cherries grown in North America.

- The fruit is bright red and about three-fourths of an inch in diameter with evergreen leaves. It grows on a large bush or small tree, usually no more than ten feet tall.

- Antioxidants abound in this fruit. Acerola is a wonderful source of vitamin C. Indeed, it is one of the highest sources in nature.

- A single acerola berry provides 80 mg of vitamin C (an entire orange has about 70 mg).

- Its high content in vitamin C is remarkable, causing it to be consumed in greater quantities in recent years. This has led to increasing economic value of the acerola fruit.

- It also appears to be a good source of the vitamin B family (niacin, riboflavin, and thiamin) and vitamin A.

- Iron, calcium, phosphorous, and potassium are also found in this versatile fruit.

- Phytonutrients are quite plentiful in acerola, including anthocyanins and flavonoid (quercetin).

The acerola is an effective neutralizer of free radicals and contains carotenoids and bioflavonoids, which provide important nutritive value and its potential use as antioxidant.

Apricot

The apricot (*Prunus armeniaca*) has been cultivated and enjoyed around the world. Many have assumed that the fruit owed its origin to the Middle East, but it was conceivably brought to that region by traders and warriors who had traveled from Europe to China and other countries of the Asian continent.

When it comes to apricots, you may be tempted to consider them as being too common to be included in any serious discussion about nutritional health. You could not be more wrong. From their beginnings in China, apricots have been used medically for centuries and still are.

- Apricots are similar to a small peach, ranging in color from dark yellow to dark orange, and grow on small trees, thirty to thirty-five feet in height.

- During World War II, American tank crews believed that apricots were bad luck and banned them from their vehicles. The superstition continues to this day.[9]

- Australian natives in the outback used the fruit as an aphrodisiac, making tea from the seed.[10]

- Research has shown that the apricot contains important antioxidants and phytonutrients.[11]

- Beta-carotene becomes vitamin A in our bodies. Apricots have a very ample supply of the antioxidants beta-carotene and lycopene.

- Moreover, phytonutrients of phenol compounds, flavonol, and anthocyanin families were shown to be present.

Apricots also provide a good supply of vitamin C and are a great source of potassium.

Aronia

The aronia (*Aronia melanocarpa*) is also known as the black chokeberry. The Native Americans and the early European settlers to America used the aronia as food. It is found in bogs and swamps.

- The fruit is black and spherical, being a small berry no more than a third of an inch in diameter.

- Aronia grows on a shrub, which usually is about three feet tall, occasionally reaching ten feet.

- When eaten alone or raw, it has a bitter taste. Clearly, the name implies that one would literally "choke" on the aronia because of its sour flavor.

- The aronia has close botanical ties to the bilberry and the cranberry in that it contains very high levels of anthocyanins and flavonoids (proanthocyanidins), among the highest of any fruit.[12]

- There are four different anthocyanins detected in aronia: proanthcyanidin, quercetin, total flavonols, and myricetin.

- Caffeic acid and its derivative are also present in relatively high concentrations and have high antioxidant activity. Also, the phenolic content of aronia is very high.

- It is likewise high in vitamin C, among other antioxidants.

Aronia's ORAC score is on par with the blueberry.

Banana

The banana (*Musa*) is a well-known fruit, grown in over one hundred countries in tropical climates. This popular fruit was first grown domestically in Southeast Asia and Australia. It was reportedly one of Alexander the Great's favorite fruits.

- The banana is found on plants from twenty to twenty-four feet tall in large "bunches." Typically, each banana is eight to ten inches in length and yellow in color.

- The USDA has found the banana to be high in antioxidants, including vitamin B_6, vitamin C, and tyramine.

- Bananas are valuable sources of potassium. These antioxidants tend to keep the LDL ("bad" cholesterol) from oxidizing and may act to prevent plaque from sticking to the walls of arteries.

Bananas also contain *protease inhibitors*, which are known to cause a thin layer of mucus to form over the stomach lining, thus protecting the stomach from developing ulcers.

Bilberry

The bilberry (*Vaccinium myrtillus*) is also known as the huckleberry, whortleberry, winberry, or myrtle blueberry. It is found in Scotland, Ireland, and some Scandinavian countries.

- This berry is tart tasting.

- The bilberry is similar in size and color to the blueberry, except the pulp is purple. Its shrub is low growing, flourishing in wet areas.

- Bilberry possesses impressive antioxidant properties. Anthocyanidins, also called anthocyanosides or anthocyanins, are abundant.

- The fruit contains about 360 mg per 100 grams of total anthocyanidins. This figure is three times higher than in black currant and more than ten times higher than amounts found in red wine.

- Studies have identified more than a dozen anthocyanidins in bilberry including delphinidin, cyanidin, petunidin, pelargonidin, peonidin, and malvidin and corresponding 3-glucosides.

Flavones and flavonols represent other flavonoid groups found in bilberry. The total content of flavonols in bilberry is 41 mg/kg, and the level of quercetin and myricetin is 89 and 20 mg/kg respectively.

Blueberry

The blueberry (*Vaccinium cyanococcus*) is a close relative of the bilberry. Blueberries are native to eastern North America but are found in South America and the South Pacific.

- Berries seldom get larger than one-third of an inch in diameter. When ripe, they are a deep indigo. They grow on shrubs from four inches to twelve feet tall.

- ADA nutritionists in a November 2003 *SELF* magazine survey named blueberries one of their top twelve must-have foods. Wild blueberries contain the highest anthocyanin levels and have the highest antioxidant capacity of any berries commercially grown in North America.

- Studies have correlated the high antioxidant activity of blueberries with their total phenolic content. The phenolic compound ellagic acid, found in blueberries, is thought to prevent or minimize the cellular damage done by free radicals, which cause cancer.

- Other blueberry phenolics include a group of compounds called *stilbenes* (resveratrol, pterostilbene, and piceatannol).

- They are packed with potassium, calcium, folic acid, and vitamins A, C, and E. Blueberries are a storehouse of fiber, and half a cup contains 2 grams of dietary fiber and only 40 calories.

- According to USDA scientists Ronald Prior and Guohua Cao, blueberries have the highest antioxidant capacity (2,400 / 100 grams) of the forty different fruits and vegetables they tested. The USDA later reported findings using the ORAC measure and ranked wild blueberries highest in antioxidant capacity per serving compared with more than twenty other fruits.

Vitamin K and tannins are also present.

Camu Camu

The camu camu (*Mycaria dubia*), like the acai palm, is another gift from the Amazon. The tree grows near water and reaches about sixteen feet in height. It has a feathery appearance.

- The camu camu fruit looks very similar to a cherry although with a reddish-purple tint. The fruit has a distinct aroma and is usually mixed with sugar or other fruits and foods.

- The camu camu has exceedingly high vitamin C content, indeed the highest of any natural product known.[13] As the world's richest source, it is said to contain thirty to sixty times more vitamin C than an orange. Oranges provide 500 to 4,000 ppm (parts per million) vitamin C; acerola has tested in the range of 16,000 to 172,000 ppm. Camu camu provides up to 500,000 ppm, or about 2 grams of vitamin C per 100 grams of fruit.

- The nutrients contained in camu camu include the amino acids serine, valine, and leucine. The fruit also contains small amounts of beta-carotene, calcium, iron, niacin, phosphorus, riboflavin, and thiamin. Alpha-pinene and d-limonene are the predominant terpenes in this fruit.

Finally, it has calcium and vitamin B_1.

Cranberry

The cranberry (*Vaccinium macrocarpon*) is well known to most of us, being a staple of Thanksgiving and Christmas celebrations in North America. In Canada, it is called the mossberry.

- Its shrub grows close to the ground, about eight inches tall or less. The cranberry seems to thrive in wet, cold bogs and swamps.

- It is red in color and rather bitter, acidic to the taste, requiring it to be sweetened or mixed with other foods.

- The cranberry is a wonderful source of antioxidants with a very acceptable ORAC score. It contains vitamin A, vitamin C, potassium, and manganese.

- The phytonutrient family polyphenols is well represented in the cranberry's pulp with ample flavonoids, anthocyanins, tannins, and petunidin. Cranberries have the highest phenolic content (measuring soluble-free and bound phenols) and antioxidant activity compared to ten other common fruits.

- The total phenol content and antioxidant activity is nearly double that of the apple, red grape, strawberry, banana, peach, lemon, orange, pear, and grapefruit.

- Cranberry juice is becoming known as a potent antibacterial for combating urinary tract infection (UTI). Contrary to popular belief, it is not the acidity of cranberry juice that provides this UTI protective effect, but rather distinct bacteria-blocking compounds called *proanthocyanidins* (PACs). While many fruits contain similar compounds, thus far only the PACs of cranberries and blueberries, which are botanically related species, have been shown to exhibit this effect.

- Cranberry's anticancer activity may come from the unique structure of its PACs. Cranberry's PACs contain a unique A-type structure, while most other fruit contains only the more common B-type PACs. This A-type structure has been shown to inhibit the proliferation of tumor cells in studies with rats.

Myricetin has been found in cranberries.

Kiwi

The kiwi (*Actinidia deliciosa*) is native to China and has had several names over the years. At least once its name was changed to avoid the taxes on the fruit![14] It has been called the Chinese gooseberry, melonette, and, most recently, the kiwifruit.

- The fruit has a fuzzy skin, is the size of a large chicken egg, and is greenish-brown in color.

- It is quite tasty and sweet. It grows on a vine similar to a grape.

- The kiwi is an excellent source of antioxidants with high levels of vitamin C and potassium.

- It also contains vitamins A and E.

- Folic acid and lutein are also present.

- Finally, the kiwi contains the phytonutrient families of flavonoids and carotenoids.

- Kiwi skews the nutritional grading curve. The health benefits of kiwifruit were so overwhelming that in 1992, the Center for Science in the Public Interest ranked kiwifruit among the top ten most nutritious fruits.

Ounce for ounce it packs more nutritional benefits than other fruits. A study conducted by Rutgers University evaluated the nutrient density of the twenty-seven most commonly consumed fruits. Nutrient density is a calculation frequently used by nutritionists to reflect a food's nutritional value. The findings rank popular fruits on the amount of value they provide per 100 grams of fruit. The study found kiwifruit, with an index of 16 (3.8 calories per nine nutrients deemed essential by the FDA) to be the most nutrient dense of all fruits.

Lychee Fruit

Also referred to as the "king of fruits" and the "symbol of romance," the lychee fruit (*Litchi chinensis*) is native to Southeast Asia. Its evergreen tree is often thirty to fifty feet tall.

- The lychee fruit is about an inch and a half in length with a diameter of an inch or so.

- Its skin is pinkish-red in hue and not edible, although the interior is off-white in color and sweet.

- Legend has it that the lychee was the favorite fruit of a Chinese emperor's No. 1 squeeze, a beautiful concubine. It is said that the emperor would order that the lychee fruit be brought to his castle by many horsemen riding fast mounts in a long relay, each leg being a short distance. Thus, the lychee has been considered a *romantic* fruit.

- The lychee is rich in vitamin C and potassium. It also contains vitamin B$_2$, riboflavin.

- Lychees have very few calories.

- The lychee fruit is filled with phytonutrients, including flavonoids, cyanidin, quercetin, the phenolic compound tannic acid, and others.

- Lychees are a good source of trace minerals and the skin is loaded with potassium.

- There are more vitamins in lychees than oranges or lemons, and they have the same dietary fiber as an apple.

- A large number of polysaccharides, which are found to have high antioxidant activity, are present in the pericarp tissues of harvested lychee fruits and should be explored as a novel potential antioxidant.

Lychee fruit pericarp (LFP) extract contains significant amounts of polyphenolic compounds and exhibits powerful antioxidative activity against fat oxidation in vitro.

Nashi Pear

The Nashi pear (*Pyrus pyrifolia*) is named for the area of China in which it was native, Nakhi (an alternative spelling of Nashi, perhaps). It has also been called the Asian pear, sand pear, and apple pear.

- The pear actually is about the size of an apple with a round shape. Nashi pears are mildly sweet and crisp to the bite.

- Nutritionally, they contain antioxidants, including vitamins C and B-complex.

- Pears also contain potassium and boron, and have a high content of lignin and pectin.

Iodine and phosphorous are also found in the Nashi pear, along with polyphenolic phytonutrients.

Passion Fruit

The passion fruit (*Passiflora edulis*) was so named by early Spanish explorers to South America. Like many other important fruits, such as the acai palm, it may also be native to the Amazon.

- The fruit's flower was thought to exhibit several symbols of the crucifixion of Christ, including His nail wounds, lash marks, crown, and three nails.

- It can grow to about the size of a grapefruit and comes in two varieties: yellow and purple. Its vine is rapidly growing and its leaves are evergreen.

- The passion fruit's flavor is somewhat tart.

- This fruit has been endowed with many phytonutrients. A partial list of its contents includes carotenoids, flavonoids (vitexin and isovitexin), hydroxycinnamic acids (scopo-letin), and alkaloids (theobromine).

- Vitamins and mineral contained in the plant are ascorbic acid, beta-carotene, calcium, iron, niacin, phosphorus, potassium, riboflavin, sodium, and thiamin.

- There is also fiber, fat, and protein contained in the passion fruit. Free amino acids in purple passion fruit juice are: arginine, aspartic acid, glycine, leucine, lysine, proline, threonine, tyrosine, and valine.

- Two passion fruits provide only 34 calories. Eaten with seeds, passion fruits are an excellent source of fiber, nearly 4 grams in two fruit servings.

Many population studies have established a link between dietary intake of the carotenoid antioxidant lycopene. Passion fruit contains a great amount of lycopene.

Pear

As we have seen earlier, the Nashi pear has been around for a long time. The typical pear you purchase in the grocery store is one of the Nashi's offspring (*Pyrus communis*).

- Pear seeds found their way into North America in the early seventeenth century by early settlers in Massachusetts.

- The pear is quite sweet. Its tree is often thirty to forty feet tall or larger.

- The fruit is usually about four inches tall and two and one-half inches in diameter.

- Pears contain vitamin C, vitamin E, and some vitamin B_2.

Phytonutrients include flavonoids (quercetin) and carotenoids (lycopene, lutein, and zeaxanthin).

Plums and Prunes

The plum (*Prunus domestica*) has a long history of consumption, dating back to the early Huns and Mongols. Pliny the Elder, the most famous Roman scientist of his day, wrote about this fruit in the first century. The plum made its appearance in America early in the eighteenth century.

- Plum trees grow to about thirty-six feet.

- The fruit is about two to three inches in diameter and purplish black in color.

- Plums range in taste from slightly tart to sweet.

- This fruit has several antioxidants, including vitamin C, vitamin B_6, and vitamin E.

- Plums also contain several phytonutrients, including hydroxycinnamic acids (scopoletin, neo-chlorogenic acid, and chlorogenic acid) and flavonoids (catechin and rutin).

- A prune is essentially a dried plum. Studies confirm that the healthful attributes of plums are multiplied when the fruit is dried to produce prunes. While fresh plums possess impressive antioxidant properties, when they are converted into prunes their antioxidant content is increased by over six times.

- Some research indicates that prunes supply the highest amounts of antioxidants of many fruits studied, fresh or dried—twice the amount found in raisins, nearly three times the amount found in blueberries, eight times the amount supplied by oranges, and nearly ten times the amount in kiwifruit.

Prunes are also a good source of fiber.

Pomegranate

The pomegranate (*Punica granatum*) is an increasingly popular fruit. Originally, it was probably native to Pakistan and Afghanistan, but it found its way to the Mediterranean before the time of Moses. It is mentioned several times in the Old Testament, and the Jews revered it and believed the pomegranate's 613 seeds represented the 613 commandments in the Torah.[15]

- The fruit is reddish in color and about two to five inches in diameter.

- The tree can range from twelve to twenty-five feet in height.

- This fruit contains vitamins C, E, and K.

- It also has an ample supply of phytonutrients, including phenolic acids such as tannins, ellagic acid, and punicalagins.

- A single medium-size pomegranate has 100 calories.

- *Tannins* are plant polyphenols that add color and a slightly tart taste to pomegranates and many other vegetables and plants.

While there are tannins in some teas and in red wine, tannins are truly abundant in pomegranate juice, which account for the juice's incredible antioxidant properties. Punicalagin is a hydrolyzable tannin that is almost exclusively found in pomegranates. This highly unique and potent polyphenol antioxidant breaks down to ellagic acid.

Purple Grape

The purple grape (*Vitis vinifera*) has been an important component of the diet of Mediterranean countries for eons. The Greeks, Egyptians, and others used it as food and for making wine for centuries before recorded history. The Greeks believed it had healing qualities. Purple grape made its initial appearance in America in the seventeenth century.

- It grows on a long vine. Each grape can be from one-half inch to one and one-fourth inches in diameter.

- The grape is sweet tasting and, as the name implies, is purple in color.

- Purple grapes are literally loaded with healthy components. They contain vitamin A, vitamin B_1, vitamin B_2, and vitamin C, along with potassium and chromium.

- Their phytonutrient complement is impressive: anthocyanins, flavonoids (catechin, kaempferol, myricetin, quercetin, proanthocyanidin, and resveratrol), and organosulfides (glutathione).

- Table grapes and wine contain many of the same polyphenols, such as resveratrol, pterostilbenes, anthocyanins, catechins, and quercetin.

- Grape juice may also be a good source of resveratrol. The predominant form of resveratrol in grapes (0.24–1.25 / C or 160 grams) and grape juice (0.17–1.07 / 5 ounces) is trans-resveratrol. Wines also contain significant amounts of resveratrol aglycones, thought to be the result of sugar cleavage during fermentation.

- Grapes contain lysozyme (muramidases), which is an antibacterial agent. Condensed tannins, complex flavonoids, pycnogenols, leucoanthocyanins, and oligomeric proanthocyanidins (OPCs) are also active constituents of grapes.

- The high phenolic content of red wine, which is about twenty to fifty times higher than white wine, is due to the incorporation of the grape skins into the fermenting grape juice during production.

- According to a the 2004 USDA database, purple grape juice made from Concord grapes tested higher in total proanthocyanidins (124 mg per 8 ounces) than any other juice or beverage it tested. Red wine had 91 mg per 5 ounces, tea had 32 mg per 8 ounces, cranberry juice had 55 mg per 8 ounces, and apple juice had 30 mg per 8 ounces. When antioxidant capacity was measured, Concord grape juice was more than two times higher than orange, apple, grapefruit, or tomato juice.

- Grape seed offers the highest concentrations of polyphenols in nature.

OPC (oligomeric proanthocyanidin), derived from grape seed, provides the most potent free-radical scavengers known with an antioxidant effect up to fifty times more potent than vitamin E and up to twenty times greater than vitamin C.

White Grape

The white grape (*Vitis vinifera*) is an almost exact match with the purple grape. Actually, it is not white but pale green. It has been used for food and wine making for centuries. Remnants of white wine were found in the tomb of the boy pharaoh of Egypt, Tutankhamen.

- Like its purple sibling, the white grape grows on a vine.

- Virtually everything we have said of the purple grape can be said of the white grape except its color and what makes the color purple.

- The same vitamins and minerals and most of the phyto-nutrients are the same for the white grape as the purple grape—except for one phytonutrient, anthocyanin. It is the presence of this compound that gives the purple grape its deep color; its absence provides for the pale green hue of the white grape.

- A genetic mutation is responsible for white grapes. A sequence of DNA is responsible for turning off the expression of the MYBA1 gene, and thus switching off pigment production in white grapes.

Flavonoids are not present in white wine because the grape skin is discarded after squeezing. Leaving the skin in the grape juice, as is done when making red wine, was found to change the color, the taste and the aroma. The skins contain the highest concentration of polyphenols, which are potent antioxidants.

Wolfberry

The wolfberry (*Lyclium chinens, Lycium barbarum*) is probably native to China and is also known as the goji berry, the boxthorn, the desert thorn, the squawberry, the "matrimony vine fruit," and the "herb of longevity."

- It is bright orange in color and oblong in shape. Its taste is sweet.

- A wolfberry grows to be one-half to one inch in length. Its plant is about three to nine feet tall. The Chinese and others have used it for medicinal purposes for more than two thousand years.

- The wolfberry is a highly nutritious plant that contains twenty-one trace minerals, copious amounts of vitamin E and vitamin C (second only to camu camu), B-complex vitamins, as well as iron. Additionally the berry is 11 to 13 percent protein, which includes nineteen amino acids (eight of which are essential for life) and the essential fatty acids, including linoleic acid.

- Bioactive polysaccharides, also called *proteoglycans*, are a family of complex carbohydrates that are bound to proteins. The *Lycium barbarum* is composed of four master polysaccharides (LBP-1, LBP-2, LBP-3, and LBP-4) that are the main active components of the wolfberry fruit.

- The wolfberry is one of the richest sources of carotenoids, including zeaxanthin.

- Wolfberry juice is unparalleled in its ability to scavenge and squelch the superoxide free radical, much like a "search and destroy" mission. According to Brunswick Laboratories, the S-ORAC of wolfberry juice is 12,200 units.

CHAPTER 8

The THREE Fs—FIBER, FRUCTOSE, and FRUIT JUICE

ARE WHOLE FRUITS BETTER THAN FRUIT JUICE? ARE CERTAIN juices better than others? To help answer these questions, in this chapter we will discuss fruits, fiber, and fructose. Then we will examine the evidence relating to fruits versus fruit juices and whether one should be preferred over the other.

Fructose, Glucose, and Sucrose: What's the Difference?

Let's start with the most important to human metabolism—glucose. Glucose is a simple sugar that is found in some plants but also in the human bloodstream, commonly referred to as "blood sugar." If there is too much in the bloodstream, it can cause a person to suffer from diabetes.

Fructose is also a simple sugar, present in fruits and their juices. In a health-conscious world, some will recoil at the mere mention of fruits because of their sugar content in the form of fructose, but you should *not* stop eating fruits because of a fear of fructose. In fact, the body needs sugars for energy. As we said in an earlier chapter, the brain has to have sugar in order to function. It is only when the body gets too much sugar too fast that health problems begin. Fruits contain fructose along with glucose, which is found in sugar cane, honey, and other sources.

The table sugar you sprinkle on your cereal, in your coffee, or use in cooking is called *sucrose*. It is also a combination of glucose and fructose. Sucrose in its simplest form is not necessarily bad for you; it's when the sugar is processed, consumed in large quantities, and your body metabolizes it that it can become detrimental to your health.

How Is Sugar Metabolized?

The process by which the body metabolizes sugar is called *glycolysis*, which is a complicated and wonderful process. Take, for example, the metabolism of one-half cup of blueberries, which like most fruits contain fructose and some glucose. When blueberries are consumed, some of their glucose is absorbed quickly by the digestive tract. The pancreas then releases insulin, allowing glucose to enter the body's cells, where it is used for energy. As we mentioned in chapter 4, this process takes place during the first fifteen minutes after the blueberries reach the small intestine.

Fructose, on the other hand, does not stimulate insulin, but it ends up in the liver and is then converted to glucose. When fructose is metabolized into glucose, which takes about fifteen to thirty minutes, insulin is again released by the pancreas and allows the newly processed glucose into the cells. So far, the body has been getting a pretty stable, level supply of glucose for about thirty to forty-five minutes.

If the blueberries were eaten whole, their fibers would have trapped some of the original glucose and fructose in their strands. The small intestine, just below the stomach, releases water, which is absorbed by the fibers and enlarges them.

While the fibers are enlarging, the sugars (fructose and glucose) are released into the blood supply and then repeat the process of glycolysis for another thirty to sixty minutes. Now the levels of glucose in the blood have been stable for a total of about sixty to ninety minutes or more.

Finally, if the blueberries were eaten with 1 percent or 2 percent milk, which contains some protein and fat, the stomach will empty more slowly into the small intestine and produce another one or two hours of rather stable glucose in the blood. This procedure minimizes the spiking of blood sugar.

What happens to your blood sugar when the fruit is squeezed into a juice instead of eaten? The length of time that the glucose levels remain stable will decrease somewhat because there is no fiber to trap the sugar until it can reach the small intestine.

This is not a serious problem for most people. However, it can be somewhat difficult for those with diabetes or for some with a prediabetic condition. Typically, drinking fruit juice during meals solves the problem, as does adding protein and a small amount of fat to your snacking while sipping fruit juices. If you are in doubt, ask your health-care provider.

Hyperglycemia and Hypoglycemia

Spikes in the amount of sugar in the body (hyperglycemia)—caused by consuming large amounts of sugar at one time—make it highly likely that you will then experience dramatically lower than normal blood sugar (hypoglycemia). This will cause subsequent hunger sooner than usual, and you may feel weak or faint without more sugar. This process can lead to obesity, since hunger leads to more food consumption and weakness tends to lead to lower activity rates.

Moreover, these spikes can also result in insulin resistance (where the insulin cannot do its job of allowing glucose into the cells), and the unwanted outcomes of diabetes, heart problems, and cancer may follow.

The Glycemic Index: A Useful Tool for Helping Identify Effects on Blood Sugar

The *glycemic index*, developed by Dr. David J. Jenkins and his associates at the University of Toronto in 1981, allows consumers to know how much spiking occurs in blood sugar as a function of the food eaten.

- If a food has a low glycemic index, sugars remain in the blood longer and at more stable levels than those identified with moderate or high glycemic indices.

- Also, the levels of insulin remain lower.

- *Remember that insulin is an inflammatory substance, so the less your body releases, the less chronic inflammation your body produces.*

Your goal: You want to keep your blood glucose levels as stable as possible, so work hard on consuming as many foods as possible with a low glycemic index.

- Most fruits, vegetables, and whole grains have a *low glycemic index*. They are considered *complex carbohydrates* because they contain both sugars and fiber.

- Candy, pancakes, table sugar, and white bread have a *high glycemic index*, while brown rice and ice cream have a *moderate glycemic index*.

The High-Fructose Corn Syrup Problem

Earlier, we mentioned the Japanese-invention of a sugar called high-fructose corn syrup (HFCS). Think of HFCS as fructose on steroids. There has been a great deal of criticism and debate over HFCS, which is used by the food manufacturing industry to sweeten everything from soft drinks to dairy products to cereal and bakery products. Some have argued that with its introduction, obesity has skyrocketed—and they are right. The HFCS itself is problematic because people are bombarded with sugar in their diets on a constant basis.

However, sugar itself is not the problem in our food consumption; the amount of sugar and other simple carbohydrate foods (white flower and white rice, for instance) that we consume are the problem.

Eating too many calories is dangerous for your health. High-fructose corn syrup makes it easy and economical for manufacturers to enhance the flavors of many foods and drinks, but it also makes it easy for you to stuff yourself with way too many calories—and quickly too.

Fiber: A Simple Step to Improving Your Health

Including fiber in your diet is one of the most intelligent nutritional steps you can take to improving your health status. Fiber comes from plants—fruits, vegetables, and nuts—but it is indigestible to humans. Grazing animals, like your friendly cow, have no trouble digesting fiber because they have an extra stomach, the rumen, in which bacteria are free to roam. These bacteria create an enzyme in the rumen of the cow or goat, and this enzyme breaks down the fiber by breaking a chemical bond, allowing the fiber to be utilized for its carbohydrate nutrients.

Humans possess no such rumen. We do have a sterile small intestine, twenty-five feet in length, in which the bacteria for breaking down fiber cannot live. Fiber just passes on through the alimentary system until it gets to the large intestine, your colon, where it is finally broken down. Once there, it is of no nutritional value since the colon is not designed to absorb the carbohydrate produced. Happily, fiber performs several important, critical functions for us.

Muscles in the small intestines squeeze and push the fiber through to its ultimate destination. In the process, energy is used and metabolism speeds up. Instead of taking some over-the-counter pill that purports to increase metabolism, why not eat more fiber-containing foods and accomplish what you really want naturally? The more fiber in your diet, the less fat is absorbed in the small intestine. Fiber actually attracts and traps some of the unwanted fats in its web and hangs on to them all the way to the colon, keeping fats from absorption by the gut. If you eat a greasy (i.e., fat-laden) cheeseburger, most of the fat ends up in your system, causing health problems. If you eat a big salad with lots of fiber, about one-third of the fat in the dressing never makes it into your system, being ushered out by the fiber.

Fiber makes your stools larger in bulk. This may sound unappealing, but the amount of pressure the intestines need to push this bulk through is less since the muscles of your intestines do not have to contract as much. Thus, hemorrhoids caused by straining and pressure are less likely to form. The colon reabsorbs water that was added earlier in the digestive process to break down carbohydrates into a nutritionally usable substance. If the transit of food is slowed, as it will be from low-fiber diets, the result is water retention, bloating, and hard, dry stools with constipation.

Your appendix is a necessary organ of your immune system, a wormlike part of the colon near the intersection of the small intestine. Constipation or slowed movement of waste matter through this area can result in inflammation of the appendix, thus creating appendicitis. Again, fiber makes this condition less likely to occur.

Look at the nutritional labeling of foods, and you will always note "calories." This can be very misleading when considering high-fiber foods. When laboratories conduct calorie estimates for foods, they do not discriminate between soluble (absorbed and nutritionally usable) carbohydrates and insoluble carbohydrates (such as fiber). Therefore, a piece of whole-wheat bread and bread from bleached white flour have the same calorie amount on the label, but the whole-wheat bread (assuming a 4-gram slice) is 12 calories less in its physiological effect on the body—the 12 calories of fiber are not digested and pass through the alimentary system. Eating more fiber-rich food really makes a dieter feel satisfied more easily.

Soluble fiber like that from beans, fruits, and oatmeal tends to enlarge when water is added, producing a sense of fullness in the stomach. Also, the food tends to stay in the stomach longer, and you feel more satisfied over a longer span of time. We noted earlier that fiber slows the release of sugars into the bloodstream and keeps the levels of insulin steadier, maintaining your blood sugar elevation. This has the sought-for outcome of decreasing hunger between meals and lowering the urge to snack and nibble. Through a complex interaction, fiber tends to increase the amount of triglycerides eliminated through the colon, reducing the level of triglycerides in the blood. There is no question that fiber is a multitasking component of good health.

Benefits of Fiber

Here are just a handful of good reasons why you should include more fiber in your diet:

- It aids in weight loss.
- It lowers fat.
- It reduces hunger and carbohydrate cravings.
- It reduces cholesterol.
- It prevents constipation.

Fiber has a salutary effect upon cholesterol levels, creating an intestinal environment that lowers the production of LDL ("bad" cholesterol). This makes a diet high in fiber content heart friendly. Also, it can aid in the dilution of bile acids that have been implicated in the instigation of cancer. To prevent the exhaustive emptying of insulin from the pancreas and thus ushering in diabetes, foods with a low-glycemic index, also known as high-fiber foods, encourage the slow rise and fall of blood sugar. Fiber also keeps the flow of bile from the gallbladder consistent, preventing stagnation, which can lead to cholecystitis (inflammation of the gallbladder) and gallstones.

We all have been told to brush our teeth after every meal. How about getting that brushing during the meal too? If you eat lots of sweets that can adhere to your teeth, those pesky little bacteria in your mouth can join with the sugar and cause cavities to form caries. Fiber can act as a toothbrush and whisk the sugar off your teeth, thus adding to the effects of your regular brushing.

The benefits of fiber are many. Suffice it to say that you need lots of it in your diet. Much of the naturally occurring fiber in your ancestors' diets was refined away to make the flour and sugar look more appealing and to dissuade pests from devouring the stored products. If even a lowly pest won't eat it, why do you have bleached white flour in your diet?

Possible Signs of Insufficient Fiber Intake

- Gas
- Bloating
- Intestinal discomfort
- Diarrhea
- Conditions such as colitis or diverticulitis

How much fiber is needed?

There is currently no recommended daily allowance (RDA) of fiber, although the daily value contained on food labels suggests 25 grams a day. The National Cancer Institute suggests you need to consume 10 to 30 grams a day. The average American gets only about 10 grams a day, well below that of our rural African brothers and sisters who ingest about 60 grams a day! To obtain maximum positive benefits from fiber, make sure you also drink plenty of water (eight 8-ounce glasses) and get regular exercise.

There are certainly conditions in which you should seek medical advice before increasing fiber content in your diet, namely colitis, chronic diarrhea, diverticulitis, heart disease, high blood pressure, intestinal bloating and discomfort, and kidney disease. Consult your physician.

Where is fiber found?

There are numerous sources of fiber. The following is a short list to help you judge your daily consumption of fiber, but it may also help you find the dietary needs unique to your tastes.[1]

	Serving size	Fiber (grams)
Breads, cereals, grains		
White bread	1 slice	0.6
Whole-grain bread	1 slice	1.7
100% All Bran	½ cup	8.8
Corn flakes	1 cup	0.7
Shredded Wheat	2 biscuits	5.5
Oatmeal, cooked	1 cup	4.0
Rice, brown, cooked	1 cup	3.5
Rice, white, cooked	⅓ cup	0.6
Fruit (fresh unless otherwise noted)		
Apple, with skin	1 large	3.3
Apricots	1	0.7
Banana	1	3.1
Blackberries	1 cup	7.6
Dates	5	3.3
Grapefruit, pink and red	½	2.0
Grapefruit, white	½	1.3
Melon, cantaloupe	1 cup	1.4
Nectarine	1	2.3
Orange	1 small	3.1
Peach	1	1.5
Pear	1 medium	5.1
Pineapple	1 cup	2.2
Plums	1 small	0.9
Prunes, dried	5	3.0

	Serving size	Fiber (grams)
Raisins	1 cup	5.4
Strawberries	1 cup	3.3
Vegetables		
Beans, baked, canned, plain	1 cup	10.4
Beans, green, cooked	1 cup	4.0
Beets, canned	1 cup	2.9
Broccoli, raw	1 cup	2.3
Cabbage, raw	1 cup	1.6
Carrots, raw	1 cup	3.1
Cauliflower, raw	1 cup	2.5
Celery, raw	1 cup	1.9
Corn, yellow, cooked	1 cup	3.9
Lentils, cooked	1 cup	15.6
Lettuce, romaine, raw	1 cup	1.2
Lettuce, iceberg, raw	1 cup	0.7
Peas, boiled	1 cup	4.5
Peas, split	1 cup	16.3
Potato, baked, fresh	½ potato	2.3
Sweet potato, cooked without skin	½ potato	3.9
Tomato, red, ripe	1 tomato	1.5
Winter squash, cooked	1 cup	5.7
Other foods		
Almonds (24 nuts)	1 oz.	3.3
Peanuts, dry roasted (approx. 28)	1 oz.	2.3
Walnuts, English (14 halves)	1 oz.	1.9

Of course, refined pasta, rice cakes, "skinless" potatoes, white bread, and white rice all have no fiber content. If the food is cooked, uncooked, chopped, mashed, or puréed, the fiber content remains the same. The positive health findings on fiber are powerful and compelling. Eat as much as you can, certainly more than the daily value of 25 grams listed on food labels. It is a valuable and simple way to enhance your health now and in the future.

Fruits vs. Fruit Juices

Are whole fruits better than juices, or vice versa? Some nutrition experts have argued that the use of fruit juices leads to weight problems and may be driving the current epidemic of obesity. They also argue that whole fruits should be preferred over 100 percent fruit juices in relationship to positive health benefits. What do the data suggest?

In a study from the United States' government database, the National Health and Nutrition Examination Survey (NHANES), researchers analyzed health information on more than seventy-five hundred children from ages two to eighteen.[2]

The findings were surprising to those who blame obesity on fruit drinks. Those children ages two to eleven years showed no difference in body mass index (BMI) between those who drank 100 percent fruit juices and those who did not.

More interesting was the discovery that those youth ages twelve to eighteen years who drank 100 percent fruit juices were significantly lower in body mass index than those who did not drink juices. The results were that fruit juices without added sugars (particularly without high-fructose corn syrup) are clearly not contributory to childhood obesity.

What about health benefits of whole fruit versus fruit juices?

In chapter 5, we described one study that demonstrated the dramatic reduction of Alzheimer's disease with the consumption of three or more fruit and vegetable juices daily.[3]

In a careful review of the research on the relative benefits of fruits and vegetables versus their 100 percent juices, scientists C. S. Ruxton, E. J. Gardner, and D. Walker concluded that whole fruits and vegetables had not been shown to be superior to their juices. They concluded that the health benefits of fruits and vegetables on cardiovascular disease and cancer was not due to the fiber in the fruits but the antioxidants and phytonutrients they contain.[4] At least in this arena, fruit juices and fruits have no obvious health benefits over one another.

Several other important findings were reported in the same review:

- One hundred percent fruit and vegetable juices reduced "bad" (LDL) cholesterol or increased "good" cholesterol.[5]

- One hundred percent fruit juices such as pomegranate and cranberry tended to raise the blood level of antioxidants.[6]

- One hundred percent fruit and vegetable juices in general had a positive impact on risk factors for heart attack.

- One hundred percent fruit and vegetable juices and whole fruits and vegetables may help reduce the risk of developing cancers.

The Scientists Concluded

When considering cancer and coronary heart disease prevention, there is no evidence that pure fruit and vegetable juices are less beneficial than whole fruit and vegetables. Thus, policies that maintain pure fruit and vegetable juices are somehow nutritionally inferior are unjustified and should be reexamined. Concerns that pure fruit and vegetable juices may impact negatively on body weight, micronutrient dilution and dental health are not borne out in the literature.[7]

Our own reviews of existing research studies are in agreement with this research review. Fruits and their 100 percent juices are essentially equivalent in their effects on our health in the realm of prevention.

For maximum benefits, make sure you include a *variety* of fruits in your juice selection.

- The more differing fruit juices, the more coverage is provided in antioxidants and phytonutrients.

- Variety is critically important because each fruit has its own array of antioxidants and phytonutrients.

- A 100 percent fruit juice blend meets all the juice requirements of taste, convenience, and nutrition.

Chances are, like most Americans, you're not consuming adequate amounts of healthy fruit and fruit juices. How can you increase your consumption to benefit your health? In the next section, we'll explore ways to optimize the health benefits of fruits and fruit juices and ways you can alter your eating habits to increase your intake of fruits.

CHAPTER 9

The QUEST for BETTER HEALTH

H UMAN BEINGS ARE ON A NEVER-ENDING QUEST TO LIVE healthier and longer lives. Ponce de Leon came to the New World with Christopher Columbus during the second expedition in 1493. In 1513, Ponce de Leon returned in command of his own expedition to find the fabled elixir contained in the Fountain of Youth, but, of course, returned to Spain empty handed. Certainly, medicine was far from a science in those days and often did more harm than good, probably killing more than its share of hapless patients via bloodletting, leaches, and purgatives.

Things began to change, slowly but surely, during the middle of the nineteenth century when physicians began using anesthetics and actually could save the lives of soldiers who had been wounded by amputating limbs and cauterizing lacerations and torn flesh. Later, surgery and trauma care became more sophisticated, along with anesthesia. Sulfa drugs and the discovery of penicillin saved more lives.

Except for an occasionally successful inoculation of infectious diseases, such as the ones that all but eradicated the dreaded smallpox (successful inoculations began as early as the late-eighteenth century) and polio (in the 1950s), prevention was not the focus of a great deal of medical energy. Most activities of researchers and practitioners were aimed at treating patients who were already suffering from illnesses or accidents. Indeed, medicine had consistently focused a great deal of its resources toward treatment and therapy.

Modern-Day Quests

Every day, research is showing us more and more benefits from fruit consumption. In previous times, research by medical and behavioral scientists was mostly conducted on small groups of "subjects" for relatively short time spans because of costs, overwhelming recordkeeping concerns, and a lack of "volunteers." Now we are beginning to see a plethora of studies on large groups of individuals conducted over long periods of time. One popular type of research design is the prospective group study in which large numbers of people (often ten thousand or more) are followed over a long time span (often three to fifteen years) and observed for the development or absence of a given disease or diseases. Well-designed studies frequently will identify several "risk factors" thought to be associated with the development of the diseases in question, such as LDL cholesterol for heart attacks, obesity for colon cancer, or race for stroke. At the end of the study, the scientist compares the rates of disease sufferers with the risk factors to determine whether the risk factors might be causally linked to the disease.

The retrospective case-controlled study is another type of research design in which individuals with a particular disease (for example, cancer of the pancreas) are evaluated on the basis of risk factors after the fact (the amount of fruit consumed on a daily basis and use of tobacco and alcohol). Epidemiological research utilizing these designs has resulted in the discovery that long-term use of fruits and fruit juices is beneficial to health in human beings. Your risks of cancer, heart disease, Alzheimer's, stroke, diabetes, and arthritis are all reduced significantly by eating fruit—lots of fruit.

Almost seven hundred thousand Americans die every year from heart disease, our leading cause of deaths.[1] Among individuals living in the developed world, there is a 73 percent reduction in new major cardiovascular disease.[2] Phytonutrients (namely, flavonoids) in fruits may impede the effects of "bad" cholesterol (LDL) by their antioxidant capabilities, preventing the cholesterol from adhering to the interiors of the blood vessels and impeding the blood flow.[3] In 2005, strokes were the third leading cause of deaths in this country,[4] and their probability decreases with the use of fruits. According to an article in *Experimental Neurology*, the anti-inflammatory and antioxidant actions of fruits may reduce the nerve cell damage and thus lower rates of debilitation and death from strokes.[5] An astounding 43 million individuals in America suffer from high blood pressure.[6] Fruit-laden diets tend to lower blood pressure.[7] Clearly, there is strong evidence that fruits in one's diet are good for the heart and blood vessels.

Cancer is the second leading cause of death in America.[8] There is strong evidence of reductions in cancer rates as a result of using copious amounts of fruit in your diet. What is it about fruits that makes them so effective in cancer prevention? Several researchers have noted possible mechanisms of their protective qualities:[9]

- Fruits interfere with the inflammatory processes at the root of most cancers (perhaps via their phytonutrients and/or antioxidants).

- Fruits can activate mechanisms that neutralize carcinogens (cancer-causing substances).

- Fruits can halt the supply of blood vessels to tumor locations, slowing down tumor formation and growth.

- Fruits can keep cells from reproducing too quickly and can aid in the destruction of previously damaged cells.

- Fruits can instigate the body's DNA repair system.

Whatever the mechanism of defense against cancer (it may be any or all of these and even other actions of fruits not yet understood), there is now evidence that you need to be eating fruit as part of your cancer-prevention regimen at any age, and the earlier the better.

Chronic Obstructive Pulmonary Disease

Chronic obstructive pulmonary disease (COPD) is the fourth leading cause of death in this country. Fifteen million of us suffer from asthma and bronchitis alone, not to mention emphysema.[10] The phytonutrients found in fruits (again, flavonoids such as quercetin) have been shown to improve lung functioning and prevent the development of COPD.[11] Vitamin C, an important antioxidant contained in many fruits, has been found in liquid on the lung surface, a great place for its antioxidant action to neutralize harmful oxidants on their way into the body.

Dietary carotenoids reduce inflammation through their antioxidant activities. Arthritis suffers have been shown to have significantly lower intakes of carotenoids than arthritis-free individuals.[12] Carotenoids and vitamin C seem to reduce the rates of arthritis. High consumers of fruits containing carotenoids have almost half as many cataracts as those with low levels of consumption.[13]

As Americans, our eating habits are dreadful. While the U.S. Department of Agriculture recommends from five to ten fruits and vegetables daily, only 17 percent of us consume two fruits a day. The average intake of fruits and vegetables daily by our population is far short of that recommended by "nutritional experts."

There are an estimated nine hundred fifty phytonutrient categories with approximately twenty-five thousand subcategories. Variety is the goal of phytonutrient utilization in the body. It is well known that overuse of one antioxidant tends to reduce the efficacy of others in the body. Phytonutrients seem to work best *en masse,* as a group working together.[14] Current thought suggests we practice eating a variety of fruits with different pigmentations to assure the phytonutrients' variety and encourage "teamwork" among them.

What about juice blends? Although some researchers have shown that fruit and fruit juice blends may have similar phytonutrient capabilities, you should include whole fruits and vegetables in your diet along with fruit blends, loading up on as many different fruits and vegetables with as large a variety of phytonutrients as possible.

Nutritional Value: Vitamins, Minerals, and Other Important Considerations

Fruits are ideal additions to one's diet, not counting the phytonutrients they contain. They tend to be mostly water, about 75 to 95 percent water![15] Thus, they are low in calorie count and good for the waistline. Of course, if sugar is added to the fruit to help maintain its shape for freezing or canning, the amount of calories goes up and up. Significant amounts of fats and protein are not found in most fruits. Avocados and ripe olives are two exceptions, containing 5 to 20 percent fat. Fruits are very good sources of fiber (with cellulose, hemicellulose, and lignin). The fiber in fruits tends to absorb water and expand into indigestible masses in the intestines, aiding in the maintenance of regular gastrointestinal functioning. (It sure sounds unappealing, but it is good for us.)

Unripened fruit contains starches, which will be altered into sugars by hydrolysis, adding water to the starch to make the sugars—sucrose, glucose, and fructose. Our parents used to say, "Never put bananas in the refrigerator." Good advice. The refrigeration of bananas keeps hydrolysis from occurring and the bananas do not ripen. Ripe fruit has more sugar than unripened fruit. You can tell by the tartness of apples or pears that they need more ripening before eating. Bruised, cooked, or peeled fruits may lose much of their vitamin load because of oxidation, which also results in rotting and spoiling.

Vitamins in General

At the turn of the twentieth century when biological science was hitting its stride, scientists became aware of vitamins. These substances were actually discovered as prevention and treatments for three illnesses: beriberi, pellagra, and scurvy. Admiral Edward Vernon of Britain's Royal Navy had years earlier given his sailors rum, water, and lime juice to ward off the dreaded scurvy, which afflicted many seamen at sea who went for months without citrus fruits.[16] As we now know, the water and rum were not functional in staving off scurvy, but probably made it more likely that the seamen would drink the concoction now known as *grog*.

The critical component in prevention was the vitamin C contained in the lime juice.

Vitamins at a Glance

- Vitamin A—promotes healthy eyes, immune system, skin, hair, and bones
- Vitamin B complex—promotes healthy brain, eyes, hair, skin, liver, and muscles
- Vitamin B_1 (thiamin)—promotes healthy brain, circulation, and digestion
- Vitamin B_2 (riboflavin)—promotes healthy cell growth, hair, nails, and skin
- Vitamin B_3 (niacin)—promotes healthy circulation, intestines, nervous system, and skin
- Vitamin B_5 (pantothenic acid)—promotes healthy adrenal gland function; helps relieve stress-related conditions such as fatigue, headaches, insomnia, depression, and anxiety
- Vitamin B_6 (pyridoxine)—promotes healthy brain function and helps to balance hormones
- Vitamin B_{12} (cobalamin)—promotes healthy nervous system and aids in digestion
- Choline (member of the B vitamin family)—promotes healthy gallbladder and liver function
- Folic acid (folate; member of the B vitamin family)—important during pregnancy; promotes healthy red blood cell formation, protein utilization, and proper cell division

Vitamins at a Glance (continued)

- Inositol (member of the B vitamin family)—promotes healthy bone marrow, eyes, and intestines; aids in lowering cholesterol and blood pressure

- Para-aminobenzoic acid (PABA; member of the B vitamin family)—promotes healthy skin, hair, and blood cell formation; supports production of vitamin B_{12}

- Vitamin C (ascorbic acid)—promotes healthy immune system; aids in formation of collagen and iron absorption

- Vitamin D (calciferol)—promotes healthy heart and thyroid; aids metabolism and assimilation of calcium for healthy bone formation

- Vitamin E (tocopherol)—promotes healthy immune system, hair, and skin (reduces scarring); reduces free radicals

- Vitamin K—promotes healthy bones and liver; aids in proper clotting of blood[17]

Back in the early 1900s, scientists thought that they had found three chemical compounds vital for health and survival that in too small amounts in the diet resulted in the three diseases. They called the substances *vitamines* (*vita* as in life, vital; and *amines*). When they discovered that not all the compounds were amines, the name was shortened to *vitamin*. At first, the vitamins all had one letter, but later it was discovered that there were a lot more than the three compounds first discovered; thus we now refer to the B vitamins (B_1, B_2, B_3, B_6, and B_{12}). Some of the original vitamins were subsequently shown to be unnecessary for human needs and removed from the list (e.g., vitamin P, pantothenic acid, and vitamin B_{17}). Others were found to be the same substance with a different name, and they too have been stricken from the list (e.g., vitamins M and X were shown to be biotin).

Vitamins are absolutely essential for life. There are now thirteen *essential* vitamins, meaning necessary for life. According to USDA researchers, from a large epidemiological study of twenty-two thousand individuals, 97 percent of our population lacks one or more essential vitamins and/or minerals.[18] Again, our eating habits are atrocious. No research to date suggests that concentrating extracts from fruits and vegetables into a pill will give you the same protection as eating the fruits or drinking their juices. Taking that multivitamin is still probably a good idea. What you may miss in your diet might be compensated with a multivitamin. But there is no substitute for fruits and fruit juices in your diet. The payoff in good health and longevity by taking both fruits and fruit blends along with vitamins and minerals in pill form awaits you down the road.

How do synthetic supplements measure up to natural vitamins? As of this printing, there is ongoing debate over this issue.

Vitamin A and beta-carotene

Cod liver oil is a traditional, natural source of vitamin A. Vitamin A is critical to the functioning of the eyes, particularly the rods and cones. A deficiency of vitamin A results in night blindness. Too much vitamin A can be toxic to the liver. Again, more is not necessarily better. It is not an antioxidant, but it stabilizes cell turnover, helping to prevent cells from reproducing too rapidly, as in cancer. Beta-carotene is a precursor to vitamin A, a so-called provitamin A. Interestingly, the body can use beta-carotene more easily than vitamin A. Too much vitamin A resulted in doubled rates of hip fractures in the elderly; not so with beta-carotene.[19] Researchers speculated that excessive vitamin A inhibited the ability of vitamin D to assist in calcium absorption. Carotenoids were originally thought quite safe in high doses; again, this is a misconception due to lack of obvious side effects and research. Recent research has shown that at higher doses (22,000 to 55,000 IUs) for five to eight years, rates of lung cancer increased from 18 to 20 percent.[20]

Vitamin C

Vitamin C is a true antioxidant and helps regenerate vitamin E in the body. Vitamin E is an antioxidant that bonds with free oxygen species. Vitamin C cleans up the bonded vitamin E and allows it to return to duty. It enhances the body's immunity system and antiviral activity. The body uses vitamin C to generate more collagen, the connective tissue that is involved in diseases such as scurvy and arthritis. Too much vitamin C has been associated with increases in kidney stones. The body cannot absorb more than 1,000 mg of vitamin C, so it has plenty of time to hang around and form oxalate for the stones. About 300 to 400 mg a day is sufficient for our nutritional needs. Some researchers have speculated that large amounts of vitamin C (in excess of 2,000 mg to 5,000 mg) may result in "clogging of brain arteries," diarrhea, and interference of cancer treatment.[21] Avoid chewable C since the ascorbic acid therein may damage the enamel. Synthetic vitamin C is most often found in the form of ascorbic acid, while citrus fruits, acerola, and rosehips provide natural sources.

Vitamin C has numerous health benefits if taken in moderation:

- Vitamin C at 300 mg daily could add six years to a person's life.[22]

- Vitamin C can reduce LDL oxidation and thus lower "bad" cholesterol.[23]

- Vitamin C can prevent the formation of cataracts with its antioxidant quality.[24]

- Vitamin C can slow the progression of rheumatoid arthritis.[25]

- Vitamin C can prevent or lessen fatigue.[26]

Folacin

The final vitamin of importance to fruit consumers is *folacin*, also known as vitamin B_9. It is found in its natural state as *folate* and synthetically as *folic acid*. Fruits containing significant amounts of folacin include papaya, cantaloupe, and navel oranges. Folate helps replicate DNA and is necessary for the development and maintenance of new cells, particularly important in the fetal stage and infancy. If an individual has a B_{12} deficiency (B_{12} is crucial for warding off anemia and for normal brain and nervous system functioning), large doses of folic acid can mask the deficiency by correcting the anemia while allowing the brain and nervous system to incur irreversible damage. If a pregnant women has too little folacin, neural tube deficiencies during pregnancy can be manifested at birth, namely spina bifida (the spinal chord is incompletely formed and the vertebrae are often open) and anencephaly (much of the skill, scalp, and brain are not formed during pregnancy). The U.S. government began requiring the fortification of some foods (e.g., pasta, bread, and flour) with folic acid in 1998 after research definitively showed that a folic acid deficiency in the diet was directly related to these problems. Since then, neural tube deficiencies have decreased. Only 40 percent of women in the child-bearing age take folic acid supplements, so much of this reduction came from fortification.[27] Additional benefits to supplementing the diet have been demonstrated:

- Folic acid reduced hypertension (high blood pressure) in females who used two and a half times (1,000 mcg) the recommended dose. Compared with those women of child-bearing age (younger than age forty-three) who consumed less than 200 mcg, the females on the larger dosage were 46 percent less likely to develop hypertension. The effect was found in women ages forty-three to seventy, but not as significant, showing an 18 percent reduction.[28]

- Folic acid may reduce the rate of decline in cognitive functioning that comes with aging. Individuals who ingested 800 mcg daily were superior on memory functioning and other cognitive measures when compared to those on placebo.[29]

- Folic acid was earlier thought to fend off heart attacks. It does lower homocysteine, implicated in heart attacks, but it now seems to offer no real protection from the heart ailments themselves.[30]

You can see from this overview of vitamins that fruits do contain beta-carotene, vitamin C, and folacin. These are very important for our overall functioning and perform vital functions for our bodies.

Minerals

Essential minerals, like essential vitamins, are necessary for life itself. Unlike vitamins, which are organic compounds (vegetable or animal in origin), minerals are inorganic. At this time, it is hard to find two people who agree on how many minerals are essential to human health and functioning. But there are two categories of minerals: macrominerals (also called essential minerals) and microminerals (also called trace minerals). The two categories are based on the amount of the mineral needed in the body, with macrominerals needed in high quantity, and microminerals needed in smaller amounts. Essential minerals cannot be used by humans unless they have been combined with another mineral or group of minerals, forming a stable salt. Table salt, NaCl, is one such salt well known to us all. There are many more. We are most often interested in the element or compound in the left side of the salt, e.g., the Na, or sodium, atom in case of table salt. The Cl, or chlorine, atom is just along for the ride to provide a neutralizing effect until the substance gets into the body.

Minerals are critical in creating enzymes in the body that act to cause or speed up chemical reactions vital for living beings. Indeed, minerals are present in every cellular reaction in the body. Once dissolved in the body, minerals (as salts) become ions (an atom or molecule with one or more electrons added or absent; thus they possess a positive or negative charge) and can be utilized by the body in this form. These metallic ions (e.g., Na, or sodium) are then placed between two identical organic ionic compounds and again are neutralized. This activity is call *chelation*. Chelation most often occurs in the gastrointestinal tract. This process provides the metallic ion with stability and protection, allowing the substance to pass through the intestinal wall and into the blood stream. Most minerals in the body are found in the chelated form. These compounds are attracted to particular tissues in the body: some find their way to the thyroid, others to the bone, and so on. For adequate chelation to occur, the mineral should be taken with a protein. Stomach enzymes and acids and certain amino acids must be present in sufficient quantity to aid in the process.

Minerals at a Glance

- Calcium—promotes healthy teeth and bones
- Copper—promotes healthy cell respiration and strong blood vessels
- Germanium—promotes healthy immune system
- Iodine—promotes healthy thyroid function
- Iron—promotes healthy circulation of oxygen in the blood
- Magnesium—promotes healthy nerves and muscles; aids in preventing headaches and irregular heartbeats
- Manganese—promotes healthy formation of enzymes, hormones, and proteins
- Molybdenum—promotes healthy kidneys and liver
- Phosphorous—promotes healthy metabolic function, bones, and teeth
- Potassium—promotes healthy cells and enzyme systems
- Selenium—promotes healthy heart, liver, and muscles
- Silica—promotes healthy arteries, hair, nails, and skin
- Sulfur—promotes healthy bones, cartilage, tendons, hair, nails, and skin
- Zinc—promotes healthy bones, eyes, kidneys, nails, skin, pancreas, prostate gland, and immune system[31]

There has been a movement in some circles to chelate minerals in the manufacturing process to make them more bioavailable; i.e., more easily used by the body. This is probably unnecessary and perhaps dangerous. As we have seen, the body already does this naturally and for free! Moreover, scientists have determined that an RDA (recommended dietary allowance) of a mineral of 1,000 mg assumes that only 300 mg are absorbed and used by the body; the rest are excreted. However, the same 1,000 mg in pre-chelated form amounts to 900 mg being absorbed. This can create an unnecessary and possibly dangerous excess. USDA researcher Jeffrey Blumberg has noted:

> Chelated minerals do not work better than non-chelated minerals. Some nutritional authorities strongly believe they are a waste of money. Although many minerals are not very bioavailable, that's actually taken into account when scientists make their mineral intake recommendations. If you are taking a supplement with the recommended amount of a mineral, you are probably getting more than enough.[32]

The essential so-called *macrominerals* (named because their RDA is greater than 200 mg/day) have been identified as follows:

- Calcium
- Chloride
- Magnesium
- Phosphorous
- Potassium
- Sodium electrolyte
- Sodium chloride
- Sulfur

The essential so-called *trace minerals* (named because their RDA is less than 200 mg/day) have been established as follows:

- Cobalt
- Copper
- Fluorine
- Iodine
- Iron

- Manganese
- Molybdenum
- Nickel
- Selenium
- Vanadium
- Zinc

Finally, there are a few other minerals that may be essential, but adequate research is lacking or contradictory:

- Bismuth
- Boron
- Chromium
- Indium
- Rubidium
- Silicon
- Titanium
- Tungsten

What about trace minerals? Are they really necessary? Should we supplement our diets with the seventy-one already identified by scientists and, unfortunately, pseudo scientists, as "essential"? Manganese, copper, lead, silver, tin, silicone, boron, and iodine have all been called essential by someone in the nutritional field, sometimes with good scientific basis but often without adequate scientific support. As with vitamins and macrominerals, their identification as *essential* occurs when a deficiency results in a clear observable physical problem in the body. The research on trace minerals has become more and more problematic with a greater appreciation for ethical treatment of research subjects. A quarter of a century ago, prisoners were used as targets of research efforts. Now, this is more and more difficult to accomplish because scientists have more stringent rules as to how humans can be accessed as guinea pigs. Much of this was made more obvious and important when it was discovered that the U.S. government had conducted studies in Tuskegee, Alabama, on syphilis with African Americans in the 1930s but failed to treat those infected even after a real cure was found with advent of antibiotic therapy, beginning with penicillin. Today, we are much more concerned with the welfare of the research participant, and rightly so.

Of course, animal research is likewise problematic and has led scientists and public health officials down dead-ends or on the proverbial "wild goose chase." Remember the great cancer scare related to saccharin? This sugar substitute, discovered in 1879, was widely used in the two World Wars when it was difficult to find good sources of sugar.[33] It was discovered in the 1950s that rats given *very high* doses of saccharin developed high rates of bladder cancer. After several years off the market, it returned (Sweet'n Low and others) with a warning label, noting that it had been shown to cause cancer in rats. Later, it was observed that rats naturally have protein in their urine (normally, humans do not), and the combination of saccharine and protein resulted in crystal formation in the rats' bladders. These glasslike crystals irritated the bladder and were causing chronic inflammation with an increase in cancer formation. Humans, unless suffering from kidney or urinary problems, do not have protein in their urine, so it was discerned that the saccharin was not capable of causing bladder cancer in humans. It is easy to overinterpret animal studies as applicable to humans, and it is often not a one-to-one match.

At this point, it is again important to note that fruits, except in a very few instances, are not great sources of trace or macrominerals. A multivitamin is easier to swallow, and you know you are getting enough of everything necessary for normal functioning of the body. Until better mechanisms of research are determined, it is probably best to avoid using trace minerals and macrominerals, since there is no adequate research to support their use. Adding untested minerals to your diet may be like playing Russian roulette with your health.

Electrolytes

Electrolytes are solutions of free ions that are critical to the body's nervous system and musculature. This means that for optimal functioning, the brain, heart, and muscles need a balance of electrolytes. Too much or too little of an electrolyte can cause serious physical problems and even death. The ions of electrolytes include potassium and calcium, among others. The Food and Drug Administration (FDA) has suggested that the addition of potassium and the reduction of sodium in our diets may significantly reduce the risks of hypertension (high blood pressure) and stroke.[34] A Canadian researcher found that regular use of orange juice raised HDL (the "good" cholesterol) by 21 percent.[35] Other fruits known to have high concentrations of potassium are figs, bananas, and avocados. Having enough potassium also aids the body in retaining nitrogen, thus increasing the mass of muscles. It is often lost in the process of sweating, but unless you are exercising at maximum performance for extended periods of time (say, six hours), not enough is lost to warrant medical replacement or supplementation. Large amounts of glucose tend to lower potassium levels, making sports drinks a poor choice of replacement since most contain sugar in copious amounts. When you lose potassium, muscles become less efficient and fatigue creeps into the body.

Individuals with certain kidney diseases can be at risk if given too much potassium and may experience cardiac arrhythmias or sudden death. This concern was highlighted when researchers discovered that one Polynesian fruit juice contained alarmingly high levels of potassium.[36] This could be dangerous for those who need to limit their potassium intake.

In the next section, we will discuss natural substances found in fruits and fruit juices that have the potential for lowering our chances of developing chronic diseases; namely, phytonutrients.

Achieving Optimum Health

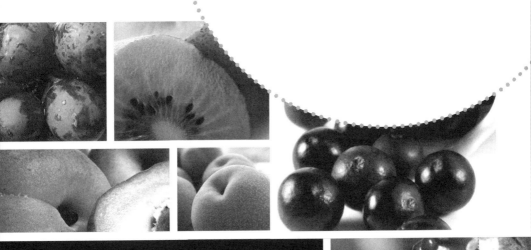

CHAPTER 10

WILD, ORGANIC, *or* CHEMICAL—DOES IT REALLY MATTER?

W E HAVE HEARD FOR DECADES THAT ORGANICALLY GROWN fruits and vegetables are better for us than conventionally grown plants. Organically grown produce represents about 1–2 percent of total food sales, with organic produce available in 73 percent of conventional grocery stores.[1] World organic food sales were an estimated $23 billion annually in 2002[2] and $40 billion in 2006.[3] Even the word *organic* conveys a sense of healthy living, clean lifestyle, and ecologically appropriate outcomes. Organic farming is compared to conventional farming in a favorable light: natural fertilizers, crop rotation, hand weeding and cultivating, and nondestructive pest control. Conventional farming with all its chemical fertilizers, herbicides, and pesticides is viewed with suspicion and disdain.

In 1990, the U.S. government got into the act and passed the Organic Foods Production Act. The act was partially what an ecologically sensitive constituency wanted, but it initially allowed *organic* to include genetic engineering, irradiation, and industrial sludge as fertilizer. By 2002, these items were eliminated for inclusion in the label *organic*. The techniques of farming allowed involved tilling and cultivating, crop rotation, use of cover crops, and fertilizing with crop waste and animal waste. There is also a national list of approved biological, botanical, or synthetic substances allowed for pest control. Only food with 95 percent of its contents organically grown could be considered organic. Those products with 70 to 90 percent organic components can be legally labeled as being *made with organic ingredients.* If a food has less than 70 percent organic substances, the use of the term *organic* can only be included in the ingredient information box on the package.[4]

Clearly, citizens of this country have a right to expect their food to be devoid of pesticides, sludge from industrial waste, and genetic engineering. Most consumers believe that *organic* foods are better for us than conventionally grown foods; they are healthier, they taste better, and they are safer and more eco-friendly. However, *there is no large body of scientific evidence that organically grown food is better for us than non-organically grown food.* Actually, there is no evidence from the scientific literature that genetic engineering, irradiation, using sludge from industrial waste, or a large variety of other practices present an unacceptable risk to humans.

What About Organic Products at the Grocery Store?

When interviewed by John Stossel on a highly controversial episode of the ABC newsmagazine *20/20,* Katherine DiMatteo of the Organic Trade Association stated, "Organic agriculture is not particularly a food safety claim. That is not what our stands are about. I think that organic agriculture and its products are healthier for the environment."[5]

Of course, almost everyone else engaged in the production, sales, and consumption of organic foods thinks more broadly. We worry about pesticides and our exposure to them. However, if the consumer washes the fruits and vegetables thoroughly before use, 99.999 percent of the pesticide residue is removed. It is the farmers and crop dusters, children of farmers, and those who are ultrasensitive to pesticides who need our concern. This in no way should diminish our vigilance regarding pesticides and their potential for harming human beings, particularly children, who as a group appear to be more sensitive to the adverse effects of herbicides, insecticides, and other pesticides. There are several childhood diseases on the rise, including asthma and brain cancers. And testicular cancers in young men are on the rise. The exact causes of these illnesses are not clear, but there is speculation among scientists that chemical pollutants are a possible culprit.

Organic farming actually may lessen the exposure of the consumer to these chemicals. However, it should be noted that even the pesticide dosing to which we are exposed in conventionally grown crops is several thousand times lower than the dangerous dosage established by U.S. government laboratories. The Food and Drug Administration monitors the levels of pesticides in our conventionally grown fruits, vegetables, and dairy products. In their latest annual report as of this printing, the FDA noted that 62.7 percent of domestic and 71.8 percent of imported foods contained no measurable pesticide levels.[6] The remaining 30 percent are almost invariably within tolerance. Even the Consumer's Union found that there were low levels of pesticides in organic foods.[7] Many of these organically produced products possessed a higher rate of bacterial contaminations than did conventionally produced products. So, the jury is still out on the issue of pesticides and herbicides.

There is some evidence, often provided by the organic food industry, that organically grown foods are healthier. These foods seem to be higher in vitamin C, phytonutrients, antioxidants, and minerals. In a head-to-head study that contrasted vitamin and mineral contact between organic and conventionally produced foods, the organic products were shown superior in the amount of studied nutrient ingredients. They were 29 percent higher in magnesium and 27 percent higher in vitamin C.[8]

Why might this be true? It is postulated that fruits grown on modern industrial farms do not have to develop defense mechanisms against predators (such as bacteria and viruses), so their levels of these mechanisms (e.g., phytonutrients and antioxidants) were lower. The farmer did all the work in defending the plants. With organic farming, more of the work is being done by the plants themselves, so they have to enhance their own defenses to survive—and we are the beneficiaries of those enhancements. However, studies conducted by unbiased laboratories have generally found no such benefits from organic foods.

Organic or Conventional—Which One Should I Choose?

There are several more considerations to remember when comparisons are made between organically produced versus conventionally produced foods. Clearly, it takes a lot more work by human beings to create organic food. More land is needed because the yields are smaller. Although many advocates of organic farming tout the better taste of such food products, blind-taste tests have found no differences. Given two fresh, ripe fruits, consumers are sometimes unable to discriminate between organic and conventional. Organically grown and cultivated plants have many more pathogens than their conventionally grown counterparts. We are all aware of the dreaded E. coli, one of the most deadly pathogens we face, which can come from manure used as fertilizer on organic farms. The original romance of organic farming seemed to emanate from the notion of the family farm. Nowadays, corporate America is rapidly taking over much of the organic farming chores.

Finally, did you know that a person can become so obsessed with the acquisition and consumption of organic foods that he or she can become diagnosable by a psychologist or other mental health professional? The condition is called *orthorexia*. Such individuals endeavor to eat perfectly. These patients spend most of their day planning meals, reading about nutrition and foods, shopping for appropriately healthy foods, and preparing meals. Because they have an unhealthy fear of accidentally eating the wrong foods and the tendency to overrate health risks inherent in foods, they may withdraw from social relationships at home and at work. Ultimately, they lose weight because they cannot find acceptable foods and thus eat a very restricted diet of so-called *health foods*. They literally worry themselves into the professionals' offices.

Deciding whether to eat organically or conventionally produced foods is clearly a personal choice with no simple solution. Either type of food production is probably safe as best we know today. Of course, most consumers are free to mix the two at their will. It probably does not make a huge difference in your overall health as long as you eat lots of fruits and vegetables and grains. However, there is a third alternative, which is just beginning to make an impact in nutritional circles—wild foods.

Wild Foods

Phytonutrients exist in all plant life. What is their function? Are they crucial to the survival of the plants? Let's revisit the discussion we had in chapter 6. Phytonutrients are natural pesticides. They work to protect plants from bacteria, viruses, molds, and fungi. The more a particular plant has to fend for itself against its natural enemies, the more powerful the phytonutrient array available. Plants increase their phytonutrient complement when subjected to assaults from the outside. So, it's not surprising to find higher amounts of phytonutrients present in organically produced fruits and vegetables as opposed to those produced by conventional methods.

But nutritionists and others are starting to believe that a third category of fruits and vegetables has even more phytonutrients: plants grown in the jungle or woods or other non-farming environments. *Wild* fruits are now being shown to have much more potent phytonutrient qualities than any farmed products, organic or conventional.

As we stated in chapter 6, once a phytonutrient is developed in a plant and you then consume it, you get the benefit of that phytochemical in much the same way as the fruit. Some, not all, of these wild fruits seem to be among the very best sources of phytonutrients, which is very important to your long-term survival and health. Whenever possible, include wild fruits in your diet. They are one huge benefit to eating fruits in general and wild fruits in particular.

The question, then, is how much are you supposed to get in your diet? We'll explore this topic, covering the various types of phytonutrients.

CHAPTER 11

HOW DO I KNOW I'M GETTING ENOUGH FRUIT?

U NFORTUNATELY, NO ONE KNOWS THE ANSWER TO THIS QUES-
tion. Allow us to explain by showing the example of lutein
and zeaxanthin. Epidemiological studies have shown positive
benefits from dietary consumption of lutein and zeaxanthin.[1] It appears
as though 6 mg/day of both compounds may be necessary to detect any
beneficial effect. It is difficult to predict from this data what the ratio
or level should be for prevention or intervention. Fruits and vegetables
are the most important dietary source of carotenoids. To date, there is
no comprehensive information on the separate content of lutein and
zeaxanthin in fruits and vegetables. Most analytical systems measure
lutein and zeaxanthin together. No government agency is responsible
for routinely testing lutein, zeaxanthin, or other dietary supplements for
their contents or quality.

What Are the Current Public Health Recommendations?

To date, no recommended dietary intake levels have been established for
lutein, zeaxanthin, and carotenoids. In an effort to set such recommendations, the Institute of Medicine at the National Academy of Sciences
reviewed the existing scientific research on carotenoids in 2000. Despite

the large body of population-based research that links high consumption of foods containing beta-carotene and other carotenoids with a reduced risk of several chronic diseases, the Institute of Medicine concluded that this evidence was not strong enough to support a required carotenoid intake level because it is not yet known if the health benefits associated with carotenoid-containing foods are due to the carotenoids or to some other substance in the food.[2]

However, the National Academy of Sciences supports the recommendations of the 2005 Dietary Guidelines for Americans, which encourages individuals to consume five or more servings of fruits and vegetables every day.[3]

Your mother was right—eating carrots may improve your eyesight. But increasing your intake of fruits and vegetables high in lutein, zeaxanthin, and carotenoids may have beneficial effects in reducing visual impairment conditions such as cataracts and macular degeneration.[4]

Good for the Eyes

Here's a partial list of fruits and vegetables high in lutein, zeaxanthin, and carotenoids:

- Dark green, leafy vegetables (spinach, kale, collard greens)
- Kiwi
- Grapes
- Oranges

The Phytonutrient Revolution

As we discussed in chapter 6, *phytonutrients*, also known as *phytochemicals*, are the secret weapons contained in fruits that account for their healing and prevention capabilities. Think of fruits as generators and warehouses of phytonutrients. There are over nine hundred groups of phytonutrients and an estimated twenty-five thousand particular types. That orange that you see in the supermarket is a great example of phyto-nutrient strength, with over one hundred seventy of them nestled in that small bundle. The orange alone has anti-inflammatory, antioxidant, and blood clot–inhibiting qualities. Since different fruits contain differing kinds of phytonutrients, variety, balance, and regular use are all impor-tant considerations.

This chapter will be more technical than the others. We want to emphasize the scientific value of fruit for maintaining good health, so we will discuss, occasionally from a scientific perspective, the nature of some of the more important phytochemicals.

Flavonoids

Flavonoids are phytonutrients found in many foods such as fruits and vegetables. Scientists have identified and named more than five thou-sand flavonoids already, and more await discovery. Everywhere in the plant kingdom, you will find these helpful *polyphenols.* A phenol is a compound in which an aromatic hydrocarbon group has a hydroxyl group attached. Phenols protect fruits and vegetables; therefore, those who eat them receive some protection from *oxidative damage.* This oxidative damage is thought to cause many if not most of the chronic illnesses from which people suffer. The phenols interfere with the devel-opment or actions of some specific enzymes in our bodies, which in turn prevent or lessen inflammation, allergies, and clotting of the blood. They are involved in lowering the levels of the angiotensin-converting enzyme (ACE) and thereby assist in lowering blood pressure. (So-called *ACE inhibitors* are medications used by physicians to lower blood pressure.) Finally, phenols can aid in the detoxification of the liver. Polyphenols are simply chains of phenols.

There has been some historical argument that flavonoids were not *bioavailable,* meaning that they did not make it into our circulatory systems. Naturally, this is of crucial importance because the ability of a substance to effect changes in our bodies may be impaired if we get very little of it. By definition, something injected into a vein is 100 percent bioavailable. This concern of non-bioavailability was based on the observation that flavonoids are most frequently attached to sugars and form glycosides, and therefore might not be capable of absorption or use by the body. Scientists now believe that many if not most of these flavonoids are indeed able to find their way into the blood supply at levels greater than previously thought possible. Clearly, they have antibacterial, antifungal, antitumor, and anti-inflammatory properties, which make them excellent dietary additions. They act as an invisible shield over blood platelets, impeding their ability to clump and clot. Finally, flavonoids seek proteins and attach themselves to them, inhibiting the development of cell multiplication and thus slowing the growth of cells that may be out of control (cancer cells, for example). This list of flavonoids' benefits is not exhaustive, but it should give you an idea as to their importance and potency.

There are six important subcategories of flavonoids that we will discuss:

1. Anthocyanins
2. Flavanols
3. Flavanones
4. Flavones
5. Flavonols
6. Isoflavones

Anthocyanins

These flavonoids consist of at least one hundred forty varieties and are found in many berries, including the acai, acerola cherries, black currants, blackberries, blueberries, cherries, pomegranates, prunes, raspberries, and strawberries, among others. Their pigments are quite beautiful with deep reds, purples, and vibrant blues. Anthocyanins are powerful anti-inflammatory substances with strong antioxidant qualities. They seem to retard the aging process by counteracting oxidative stress found in aging bodies (which are known to produce less anti-inflammatory substances as we grow older). They can reduce the damage caused by "bad" (LDL) cholesterol and may in turn prevent atherosclerosis, or hardening of the arteries. Anthocyanins appear to relax our blood vessels and lower blood pressure in addition to preventing blood clotting. They also reduce the ability of blood vessels to service cancer cells with nutrition by lowering the ability of vessels to reach tumor sites. They may aid in restoration of the heart rhythm, making the heart more responsive to the requirements of exercise and activity. They work against the development of diabetes in adults via several mechanisms, such as reducing blood sugar and vessel damage, while, perhaps, increasing the rate of insulin production. There are claims that anthocyanins reduce the formation of *tyrosine nitration*, which is associated with several diseases of the nervous system.

Because these anthocyanins degrade rapidly when the fruit is harvested (about half of their levels are gone within forty-eight hours), they must be protected. Often, produce farmers and processors use citric acid to protect the anthocyanins from such degradation.

Flavanols

The most important flavanols are *catechins*. Catechins are found in several fruits, including apples, cranberries, currants, grapes, and peaches. These flavanols have a strong antioxidant and anti-inflammatory capabilities. They seem to interfere with the oxidative changes caused by free radicals interacting with "bad" cholesterol, which results in atherosclerosis, or hardening of the arterial walls, thus possibly preventing some strokes and heart attacks. Catechins also have been shown to neutralize free radicals. These flavanols also inhibit the proliferation of cancer cells, helping prevent their spread (metastases). They lower the amount of glucose (sugar) absorbed in the small intestine and may aid in the prevention of diabetes. Finally, catechins may stop the formation of blood vessels (angiogenesis) that supply nutrients to cancerous tumors.

Flavanones

Flavanones are commonly known as *bioflavonoids* in the popular media. There are four kinds of flavanones: hesperidin, rutin, naringenin, and eriodictin. When you hear of bioflavonoids, you probably think about citrus fruits, and you would be correct. Flavanones are found in grapefruit, lemons, limes, oranges, and tangerines. Other fruits are also good sources of flavanones, including apricots, bilberries, cherries, grapes, and prunes. Flavanones, potent antioxidants, along with vitamin C were originally thought to be a single substance responsible for preventing scurvy—citrin—until separated chemically by Nobel Prize–winner Albert Szent-Gyorgyi in the 1930s. Indeed, the flavanones were originally called vitamin P because they were shown to prevent the leakage of blood from small vessels, our capillaries. They decreased *permeability*, thus the moniker vitamin P.

Flavanones actually aid in the body's use of vitamin C, slowing down its absorption and allowing this important vitamin to remain in the blood supply for longer periods of time. If you eat the whole fruit (less the skin), you will get enough of both. Flavanones also assist in preventing the harmful buildup of iron in the blood while vitamin C aids in the absorption of iron. Balance again is an important and ever-present component of good health.

Flavanones are also important in the breaking down of *fibrin*, an important aspect of blood clotting and subsequent inflammation. They can reduce spider veins and prevent varicose veins along with hemorrhoids and the rupture of vessels in the eyes of diabetics. Flavanones have the ability to remove viruses from the blood. They seem particularly adept at preventing problems of circulation and may indeed be protective of cardiovascular disease in general.

Flavones

As with the other phenols, flavones have two types, apigenin and luteolin. They are found mainly in olives. Since olives are not fruit, we will not discuss them further except to note that they should be included as part of a balanced diet.

Flavonols

There are two important classes of flavonols: quercetin and myricetin. Quercetin is found in green apple skins, cherries, cranberries, red grapes, sea buckthorn, strawberries, and tomatoes. Quercetin is a complex carbohydrate when found in fruits, meaning that it has three or more sugar molecules attached. It has many excellent health-related properties, including antiviral and antibacterial functions. Quercetin can inhibit the multiplication of the bacteria that cause peptic ulcers, *helicobacter pylori*. Moreover, it impedes the growth of the *herpes* virus and the virus responsible for mononucleosis, *Epstein-Barr*. Quercetin also lowers the accumulation of sorbitol in diabetics, thought to be responsible for kidney and nerve damage. It lowers inflammatory processes in the body, particularly in the blood vessels, so it helps prevent heart attacks. Quercetin inhibits the growth of cancers and their metastases (the spread of cancerous cells around the body). An apple a day may indeed keep the doctor away!

Keep the Doctor Away With an Apple a Day!

One study showed that women who regularly ate apples had a 13 to 22 percent decrease in risk of cardiovascular disease.[5]

Myricetin can be found in bilberries, black currants, blueberries, and cranberries. It appears to have strong anti-inflammatory and antioxidant capabilities and may aid in neutralizing the "bad" cholesterol, LDL. Myricetin may reduce the formation of cancer cells and also slow the development of arterial narrowing, a precursor to heart attacks and strokes.

Isoflavones

Isoflavones are also known as *phytoestrogens* and have several subtypes, including daidzein, enterolactone, equol, genistein, and lignins. Isoflavones are found in berries and a few other fruits. As the name *phytoestrogens* implies, they act in a manner similar to the female hormone estrogen. They are considered strong antioxidants and may impede those enzymes that stimulate some cancers. They appear to have tumor-suppressing capabilities and may prevent bone loss (osteoporosis) and lower "bad" (LDL) cholesterol.

Non-Flavonoid Polyphenols

To complement the flavonoid family of polyphenols is the non-flavonoid polyphenol family, or simply *phenolic acids*, which include:

- Caffeic acid
- Chlorogenic acid
- Cinnamic acid
- Egallic acid
- Ferulic acid
- Neochlorogenic acid

Caffeic acid

Caffeic acid is found in blueberries, grapes, prunes, and grains. It acts as a strong antioxidant. It has antimetastatic properties along with the possibility of inhibiting the development of cancers; thus it may prevent the growth and spread of cancers. Caffeic acid appears to protect against heart attacks by reducing the clumping together of platelets. Finally, a substance named 5-lipoxygenase (5LOX) has been shown to create inflammation by metabolizing arachidonic acid from our diets and forming leukotrienes. Caffeic acid has been shown to interfere with this formation and may result in lowering inflammation.

In conclusion

As you can tell from the discussions about just a few of the phytonutrients, these compounds perform many health maintenance functions. One could write many more pages on the various phytochemicals and still not exhaust the massive volume of research regarding the types of these substances and their benefits. Space does not allow us to detail the effects of chlorogenic acid, cinnamic acid, egallic acid, ferulic acid, and neochlorogenic acid, not to mention a huge number of others. Nonetheless, we believe you needed to understand that each phytonutrient performs an important role or roles in keeping us healthy. Since no single substance can perform all the roles, we need to consume a wide variety of these phytochemicals by eating lots of different fruits and drinking the juices of many fruits.

Magic Pills, Miracle Drugs, and Snake-Oil Salesmen

Marketers and distributors of natural products are not permitted to talk in terms of dosage. When they do, this raises a red flag for the FDA to accuse them of selling a drug, which would be illegal. A dosage implies it has clinically proven value, is used for the treatment, prevention, or cure of a disease, or has been clinically proven to mitigate symptoms. There are only about a dozen foods and supplements about which such claims can be made (e.g., oats, soy, psyllium, omega-3 fatty acids, calcium, and folic acid) in a health-food industry with over one hundred thousand products and billions in profits ($17 billion). The nature of food is restorative and cumulative and easier to think in terms of servings, which in the case of juice is 4 to 6 ounces or a medium-sized fruit.

Strive to eat a variety of different colors because your body needs a variety of phytochemicals—the darker the color, the more concentrated the amounts of phytochemicals. Do not try to single out a few magic vitamins, antioxidants, or phytochemicals to take as supplements. Instead of emphasizing a particular fruit, eat a wide variety in generous quantities every day. Antioxidants tend to work as a team in synergistic fashion. Some of these antioxidants may not have relevant biological activity on their own, and they do not work through identical biochemical mechanisms. Foods contain phytonutrients in combination, and it could be the unique mixture that is key to their effectiveness. It is one of the most important favors you can do yourself, and the benefits are well backed by research. That is why nutritionists no longer stress individual nutrients or phytonutrients, but instead they promote a plant-based diet of fruits and vegetables. Fruits should be chosen based on their traditional-based healing values as well as their specific health benefits and unique phyto-nutrient composition validated by modern science.

Foods serve as supplements to complement a healthy way of life. People cannot claim that foods prevent or cure any malady. These are natural products designed to supply and restore your body to optimal state. They work synergistically and in harmony to bring about balance in your body. Hopefully, you have absorbed that notion into your brain and are ready to turn over a new leaf to implement a healthier way of life. In the next chapter, we'll give you a few tips on how to get in the habit of making better food choices, and we'll show you one patient's journey to optimum health.

CHAPTER 12

GET INTO *the* HABIT!

W E HAVE PRESENTED IN SOME DETAIL THE CASE FOR EATING more fruits and drinking more 100 percent fruit juices. Based upon the scientific research reviewed in this book, it is clear that fruits and fruit juices should be an integral and continuous part of your diet!

Developing a healthy diet has been shown to increase health and vitality and reduce the chances of developing chronic illnesses. Unfortunately, the fact that so many do not consume enough of these nutritious foods is of particular concern.

What can be done to increase the consumption of fruits and fruit juices? In this final chapter, we will present some principles of behavior change and how they apply to altering your own eating habits.

Law of Reinforcement

Your parents and grandparents intuitively knew how to change your behavior. There were consequences for the behaviors they wanted to increase in frequency and different consequences for those behaviors they wanted to decrease in frequency.

For example:

- You were not allowed to go on that date unless your room was clean.

- If you came home late, you were not allowed driving privileges for a week.

- If you ate your spinach, you were given dessert.

- If you talked back, you were sent to your room.

The law of reinforcement fits these examples perfectly and represents a very useful rule for changing behavior: whatever occurs or fails to occur *immediately after a behavior* determines whether it will be repeated.

This law of behavior change is very important to consider when altering your own habit pattern. It operates in many areas of our lives. (For example, the seat belt buzzers in automobiles sound off if you fail to buckle up.)

Remember that most of our undesirable behaviors do not change as a result of reason or logic. If logic worked on behavior change, no one would use tobacco, drink too much, eat too much, or lead a sedentary lifestyle. Everyone would consume seven to eleven fruits and vegetables every day. Talk is cheap, goes the old saying. But talk doesn't work very well. *What you must change is consequences.* It is not a lecture or logical treatise that will work. It is rewarding or punishing the targeted behavior that will help change its frequency.*

Therefore, to change what you eat, set up a behavior change program using the following steps:

1. Specify the behavior you wish to change.

2. Measure how often you currently perform the behavior.

3. Identify possible motivators.

4. Develop a program for change based upon the law of reinforcement.

5. Measure again to see if your program for change worked.

---

* For more information, please read *Positive Parenting* by Roger C. Rinn and Allan Markle (Research Media, 1977).

Five Steps of Behavior Change

How can you use these behavior change steps to increase the number of fruits and fruit juices you consume every day? Follow these steps.

First, *specify* how many fruits, fruit juices, and vegetables you wish to consume every day. Be specific about when you'll eat them—at breakfast, lunch, dinner, or snack.

Second, *measure* how many you are currently eating by keeping a food log for a week. This will be your baseline to evaluate whether the program you develop will be effective.

Third, *identify* some motivators. There are three types: material, social, and activity. Material motivators might include money, clothing, video games, or a set of weights, for example. Social motivators include praise from others and approval from significant others. Activity motivators include exercise, sports, movies, television viewing, and reading.

Fourth, *develop* a program for change by rewarding yourself when you consume the desired number of fruits, fruit juices, and vegetables each meal.

Measure your progress and make certain to reward yourself *immediately* after you perform the desired behavior. You can design your own program. Be careful to make most of your rewards as immediate as possible.

As an example, here's a program developed by one of our patients.

One Patient's Program

This patient limited her red meat, used olive oil in cooking, ate very little sugar, drank skim milk, and consumed whole wheat and oats. She needed to increase her fruits, fruit juices, and vegetable intake. Here's how she applied the five steps of behavior change.

1. **Specify**: breakfast, one fruit and one 100 percent fruit juice; lunch, two fruits, one 100 percent fruit juice, and one vegetable; dinner, two fruits, one 100 percent fruit juice, and two vegetables

2. **Measure**: Over seven days, she averaged only 2.4 fruits or vegetables daily.

3. **Identify**: Walking with husband after lunch; reading novels in the evening after dinner

4. **Develop**: Every day that Barbara consumed the target number of fruits, fruit juices, and vegetables at breakfast and lunch, her husband would walk with her for forty-five minutes from 12:45 p.m. until 1:30 p.m. Every day that Barbara consumed the target number of fruits, fruit juices, and vegetables at all three meals, her husband would wash the dishes and she would read a novel for one hour.

5. **Measure**: After two weeks on the program, Barbara averaged 6.8 fruits, fruit juices, and vegetables daily. After four weeks, she was consuming an average of 10.7 daily. Finally, after six weeks, she was averaging almost 11 fruits, fruit juices, and vegetables daily!

Not all programs work as nicely as Barbara's. Her husband was a great help, and through their teamwork, she reached her goal. If your program hits a snag, change it! Remember to eat the fruit first, and follow consumption by a reward.

Variety Is the Spice of Life!

There are compelling reasons to consider 100 percent fruit juices as a regular part of your daily food intake.

- They are handy and easy to store at your home or place of work.

- You can use juices as snacks midmornings and afternoons.

- The more convenient a food is to use, the more likely you are to consume it.

- The tastier a food is, the more likely you are to want it.

- The more nutritious a food is, the more likely your body is to need it.

- Replace that soft drink, regular or diet, with a 100 percent fruit juice.

Make sure you include a *variety* of fruits in your juice selection.

- The more differing fruit juices, the more coverage is provided in antioxidants and phytonutrients.

- Variety is critically important because each fruit has its own array of antioxidants and phytonutrients (as we have seen earlier in this book).

- A 100 percent fruit juice blend meets all the juice requirements of taste, convenience, and nutrition.

How can you keep your focus on health and proper diet?

- Surround yourself with like-minded friends and companions.

- Join a health club or gym and exercise regularly.

- Talk about illness prevention, and tell those who will reward you with praise and approval all about your current successes in changing your lifestyle to a health-friendly focus. It is totally appropriate to brag on your own efforts.

- Find an array of fruit juices or a single blend that appeals to your taste and drink it.

A Final Note

It is never too late to start taking care of yourself. Drinking more 100 percent fruit juices and eating more fruits and vegetables can help you begin the journey to a healthy tomorrow, but you have to start today!

SUPER FRUITS—MYTH, MIRACLE, *or* MALARKEY?

F RUITS SEEM TO HAVE HAD A MYSTICAL HEALING QUALITY throughout history, and the folklore of many cultures bears this out. There has long been a strong reception in the medicinal value of fruits far back in recorded history. Each culture had its favorites. Despite years of use of fruits for prevention and treatment of disease and dysfunction, there has been scant research until recent times as to their actual effectiveness.

The healing effects of the *wolfberry* has been extolled in the written word for over three thousand years. The wolfberry was originally found in the Ningxia Province of China. Legend and rumor have supposed that the inhabitants of this province lived long lives, perhaps one hundred fifty years in some cases. The Himalayan Hunzukuts likewise have eaten the wolfberry for centuries with similar claims of great strength, endurance, and longevity. Legend has it that wolfberries fell into a well frequented by Buddhist monks, and when they drank from the waters, they would not lose their teeth or the pigment in their hair. It is now a very popular fruit worldwide.

The *aronia* or black chokeberry is very similar to the cranberry. It was originally found growing wild in eastern North America and was popular for its alleged medicinal qualities. Native Americans and pilgrims thought aronia had healing capabilities due to the extremely bitter taste of the berries. They observed that birds feasted on them and did not die, but birds have no sense of "bitter." It was undoubtedly a big surprise to an unwary person when he or she bit into the tasty-looking berry and discovered its bitter flavor: "If it tastes bad and doesn't kill you, it must be medicine." On scientific assay, it has been shown to have high antioxidant capabilities.[1]

Kiwi or *kiwifruit* was first found in southern China and was originally called the Chinese gooseberry. It found its way to New Zealand and was subsequently renamed by an entrepreneur after the kiwi, a non-flying national bird of New Zealand. Chinese medical practitioners used the kiwi before the dawn of recorded history to treat a large variety of aches, pains, and ailments.

The *mangosteen,* goes the fable, was coveted by Queen Victoria, who offered a prize to anyone who could provide her with a taste. Found originally in Southeast Asia, the fruit was thought by the ancients to possess great healing qualities. Even early Europeans thought it was a powerful healing fruit. Surprisingly, it has not been shown to be particularly well endowed with antioxidants and other health-enhancing substances.

During World War II, Royal Air Force pilots discovered serendipitously that the *bilberry* seemed to improve their night vision since their night bombing successes improved dramatically. Sadly, this was not found to be the great miracle as touted by those intrepid flyers. Instead, they were probably successful because of a top-secret invention at that time, radar, which aided in pinpointing their bombing runs. Subsequent research has not shown any significant improvement in the night vision of those using bilberry. Long before its current use, it was thought to improve gastrointestinal disorders and discomfort, being made into a salve and placed on the stomach of the sufferer.

The *acai berry* has been used as part of the regular diet of at least three indigenous tribes of Brazil in the rain forest, providing up to two-fifths of their food by weight![2] It is plentiful in Brazil and parts of Peru. The regional folklore describes the acai berry as providing incredible energy to its users, very important for survival in a hostile environment with enemy warriors a constant concern. The local Brazilians eat it regularly and attribute to it great healing qualities, stopping tooth decay, treating skin diseases, and preventing illnesses in general. There are a number of studies suggesting that the acai berry is indeed rich in antioxidants, fats, proteins, and carbohydrates.[3] Other research has shown that the acai is filled with abundant phytonutrients.[4]

The *noni* or *Indian mulberry* is native to Southeast Asia and now is found around the South Pacific, including Tahiti and Hawaii. It has a long history of use as treatment for just about everything you can conjure, including asthma, dysentery, headache, menstrual cramps, stomach upsets, and pain.

When the Spanish conquistadores explored the South American continent, they discovered the *passion fruit,* so named by their Catholic priests who saw a large number of religious symbols on and about the fruit, including the crucifixion, a crown of thorns, stigmata, and other symbols of Christ's passion. The fruit is thought to have many health attributes. In Puerto Rico, the passion fruit is thought to lower blood pressure. In South America, its leaves are thought to possess a tranquilizing effect to counteract agitation.

The *cranberry* is a Thanksgiving fruit and has been popular naturopathic treatment for urinary tract infections (UTIs) for a century. Cranberries seem to make it very difficult for bacteria to attach to the lining of the bladder itself. The Native Americans used the cranberries for food and gave them to starving Pilgrims; thus cranberries became a staple of the holiday. Not surprisingly, cranberries are very rich in phytonutrients.

Well, What Is It?

We have provided a very cursory overview of fruits to show that a lot of what we think we know from history and popular culture about fruits is a little bit of all three: myth, miracle, and malarkey. Just because a fruit or vegetable was deemed health promoting by an earlier culture does not mean much. People assert a lot of beliefs about foods that later are found to be false. Even Galen, the great Roman physician of antiquity, admonished his followers to eschew fruits altogether, asserting that they were harmful. Other cultures and times seem to have gotten it wrong more often than not. More and more, we have discovered that fruits are indeed crucial components of a healthy lifestyle, but often not in the way the myths of old would lead us to believe. Our ancestors did not know about phytonutrients, essential fatty acids, and other health-promoting components of fruits and other foods.

Some fruits and fruit juices are being marketed with incredible claims of "life enhancement" and "ultimate health." Many of the juice products and juice blends tend to share a common theme. They are the "first and only" product to contain a particular fruit. They give the users of the product a "cure" for what ails them. They are a "miracle." *Certainly, avoid any product that claims curative features.* There is no evidence that fruit *cures* cancer. There is no evidence that fruit juices *cure* diabetes or coronary artery disease. Otherwise, fruits and fruit juices would be sold as drugs. They are not drugs. They are food. They do seem to be associated with better health outcomes, and the current spate of research in the preventive qualities of fruit and fruit juice points strongly in the direction of illness prevention. However, this research is only in its infancy.

Obviously, based upon current science, we believe that some fruit juices can be more helpful than others. We do not believe that any of the juice products or juice blends on the market today are necessarily "bad" for you. Indeed, some appear to have great health benefits. What we do provide is a way of looking at them and understanding what they can do for your overall health needs. We want to make you an informed consumer of fruits and fruit juices.

Consume more fruit. Drink more 100 percent fruit blends. Harness the healing power of fruit today!

FRUIT RECIPES

Great-Tasting Juice Combos

For any of the following juice combos, process fruit in a juicer or blender and serve in tall glass with ice. Unless otherwise indicated, all recipes provide a single serving.

Options:

- Sweeten any of the following with honey or agave nectar to taste.

- Turn any of the following juice combos into smoothies by adding ½ cup of plain yogurt or ½ cup of ice to the blender.

Apricot-Pear Juice

2 apricots (or peaches), sliced
2 pears, sliced (or 1 apple and 1 pear, sliced)

Aronia-Apple Juice

2 cups aronia berries
2 apples, cored and sliced

Blueberry-Acerola Juice

1 cup acerola berries (or cherries)
1 cup blueberries (or bilberries)
1 pear (or apple), sliced

Cranberry-Orange Juice

2 cups cranberries
2 oranges, peeled and sectioned

Passion Fruit-Lemon Juice

3 passion fruit (scoop fruit out of rind and discard rind)
1 lemon, peeled and sectioned (remove seeds)
1 Tbsp. chopped fresh mint leaves

Plum-Strawberry-Peach Juice

1 plum, sliced
1 cup strawberries, sliced
1 peach, sliced

Pomegranate-Camu Camu Juice

1 cup extracted pomegranate kernels
1 cup strawberries
½ cup camu camu berries
Freshly grated ginger to taste (try ½ tsp. to start)

Tip for extracting pomegranate kernels: Score the pomegranate into sections and soak in a bowl of water for five minutes. Break open the sections in the water and allow the kernels to separate from the rind and sink to the bottom of the water. Discard rind and drain kernels in colander.

Other Fruit Recipes

Acai-Banana Smoothie

1 cup acai berries
1 banana, sliced
½ cup plain yogurt
1 tsp. granola (optional)

Combine fruit and yogurt in blender. Serve in tall glass and top with granola (optional).

Optional: Add strawberry, raspberry, or blueberry to taste.

Fruit Punch

2 oranges, peeled and sectioned
4 pears, cored and sliced
24 strawberries, stems removed
24–32 oz. sparkling mineral water

Combine fruit in a juicer or blender. Pour into four tall glasses. Add sparkling water and ice to each glass and serve.

Homemade Ginger Ale

1 Nashi pear (or apple), cored and sliced
Freshly grated ginger to taste (try ½ tsp. to start)
½ lime, peeled and sectioned
½ lemon, peeled and sectioned (remove seeds)
1 cup white grapes (or purple grapes)
6–8 oz. sparkling mineral water

In juicer or blender, combine fruit and ginger until well mixed. Pour juice in a tall glass; add ice and sparkling water.

Substitution: You may substitute jarred pre-minced ginger for fresh ginger.

Rainbow Fruit Salad

2–3 lychees, peeled and cubed
1 papaya (or mango), peeled and cubed
1 honeydew (or cantaloupe), cubed
3–4 bananas, sliced
5 kiwis, peeled and sliced
6–8 apricots (or peaches), sliced
2 cups grapes (white or purple)
2 cups blueberries (or bilberries)
2 cups sliced strawberries
½ cup dried wolfberries
2–3 tsp. vanilla
Honey or agave nectar to taste (optional)

Combine fruit in large bowl and sweeten with vanilla, honey, or agave to taste.

Options:

- You may use canned apricots or peaches instead of fresh fruit. If you add the syrup from the canned fruit to the salad, no honey or agave will be needed.

- Process leftover fruit salad into smoothies by combining in a blender with plain yogurt or ice.

Tropical Delight

1 mango, peeled and sliced
1 orange, peeled and sectioned
1 kiwi, peeled and sliced
6–8 oz. sparkling mineral water

In juicer or blender, combine fruits until well blended. Pour into tall glass. Add sparkling water and ice.

NOTES

Chapter 1
Trouble in Paradise

1. NationMaster.com, "Health Statistics: Life Expectancy," http://www
.nationmaster.com/graph/hea_lif_exp_hea_yea-health-life-expectancy-healthy-
years (accessed July 6, 2008).

2. Chris L. Peterson and Rachel Burton, "U.S. Health Care Spending:
Comparison with Other OECD Countries," CRS Report for Congress, September
17, 2007, http://assets.opencrs.com/rpts/RL34175_20070917.pdf (accessed July 6,
2008).

3. Bureau of Labor Education, University of Maine, "The U.S. Health Care
System: Best in the World, or Just the Most Expensive," Summer 2001, http://dll
.umaine.edu/ble/U.S.%20HCweb.pdf (accessed July 6, 2008).

4. John Steen, director, Community Health Planning, Columbus (OH) Health
Department "With Liberty and Justice for All?" August 2000, http://www
.ahpanet.org/files/With%20Liberty%20and%20Justice%20for%20All.pdf (accessed
July 6, 2008).

5. Harvard School of Public Health, "The Nutrition Source: Healthy Eating
Pyramid," http://www.hsph.harvard.edu/nutritionsource/what-should-you-eat/
pyramid/ (accessed July 14, 2008).

6. H. M. Blanck et al., "Fruit and Vegetable Consumption Among Adults—
United States, 2005," *Morbidity and Mortality Weekly Report 56*, no. 10 (March
16, 2007): 213–217, http://www.cdc.gov/mmwr/preview/mmwrhtml/mm5610a2
.htm (accessed July 6, 2008).

7. P. P. Basiotis et al., "Consumption of Food Group Servings: People's
Perceptions vs. Reality," *Nutrition Insights*, October 2000, http://www.cnpp.usda
.gov/Publications/NutritionInsights/Insight20.pdf (accessed July 6, 2008).

Chapter 2
Inflammation—the Body's SWAT Team

1. J. Walston et al., "Frailty and Activation of the Inflammation and Coagulation Systems With and Without Clinical Comorbidities," *Archives of Internal Medicine* 162 (2002): 2333–2341.

2. U.S. Department of Agriculture, "USDA Dietary Guidelines for Americans 2005, From the Executive Summary," http://www.health.gov/dietaryguidelines/ dga2005/document/html/executivesummary.htm (accessed July 4, 2008).

3. Centers for Disease Control and Prevention, "Defining Overweight and Obesity, http://www.cdc.gov/nccdphp/dnpa/obesity/defining.htm (accessed July 7, 2008).

4. Breastcancer,org, "Abnormal Breast Cancer Genes," http://www.breastcancer .org/risk/genetic/new_research/20050428.jsp (accessed July 5, 2008); E. Claus et al., "Abnormal Breast Cancer Genes Are as Common in Women with DCIS as in Women with Invasive Breast Cancer," *Journal of the American Medical Association* (February 23, 2005).

5. G. Danaei et al., "Causes of Cancer in the World: Comparative Risk Assessment of Nine Behavioural and Environmental Risk Factors," *Lancet* 366, no. 9499 (November 19, 2005): 1784–1793.

6. Ibid.

7. American Institute for Cancer Research, "Eat More of a Variety of Vegetables, Fruits, Whole Grains, and Legumes, Such as Beans," http://www.aicr.org/site/ PageServer?pagename=dc_recs_04_variety_of_vegetables (accessed July 23, 2008).

8. Carrie H. S. Ruxton, Elaine J. Gardner, and Drew Walker, "Can Pure Fruit and Vegetable Juices Protect Against Cancer and Cardiovascular Disease Too? A Review of the Evidence," *International Journal of Food Sciences and Nutrition* 57 (May 2006): 249–272.

9. National Heart Lung and Blood Institute, "What Are the Signs and Symptoms of Carotid Artery Disease," http://www.nhlbi.nih.gov/health/dci/ Diseases/catd/catd_signsandsymptoms.html (accessed July 5, 2008).

10. "Pain Takes a Holiday," e-Alert, September 8, 2003, as quoted in Health Sciences Institute, "Aspirin and Heart Attacks: Double-Edged Wonder," http:// www.hsibaltimore.com/ealerts/ea200407/ea20040714.html (accessed July 7, 2008).

Chapter 3
Bringing the Body Into Balance

1. Martin E. P. Seligman et al., *Learned Helplessness* (n.p.: Oxford University Press USA, 1995), 20.

2. Martin E. P. Seligman, *Learned Optimism* (n.p.: Vintage, 2006).

Chapter 4
Dietary Secrets of the Past

1. ScienceDaily.com, "160,000-year-old Fossilized Skulls From Ethiopia Are Oldest Modern Humans," June 12, 2003, http://www.sciencedaily.com/releases/2003/06/030612090827.htm (accessed July 23, 2008).

2. C. J. Lewis et al., "Nutrient Intakes and Body Weights of Persons Consuming High and Moderate Levels of Added Sugars," *Journal of the American Dietetic Association* 92 (1992): 708–713.

3. M. K. Lockwood and C. D. Eckhert, "Sucrose-induced Lipid, Glucose, and Insulin Elevations, Microvascular Injury, and Selenium," *Am J Physiol Regul Integr Comp Physiol* 262 (1992): R144–R149, http://ajpregu.physiology.org/cgi/content/abstract/262/1/R144 (accessed July 23, 2008).

4. Lorraine H. Marchand, "The Pima Indians: Obesity and Diabetes," National Institute of Diabetes and Digestive and Kidney Diseases, http://diabetes.niddk.nih.gov/dm/pubs/pima/obesity/obesity.htm (accessed July 23, 2008).

5. James H. Dickson et al, "Kwäday Dän Ts'ìnchì, the First Ancient Body of a Man From a North American Glacier: Reconstructing His Last Days by Intestinal and Biomolecular Analyses," *The Holocene* 14, no. 4 (May 2004): 481–486, http://hol.sagepub.com/cgi/content/abstract/14/4/481 (accessed July 9, 2008).

6. Gary Taubes, "The Epidemic That Wasn't?" *Science* 291 (March 30, 2001): 2540, http://www.sciencemag.org/cgi/content/summary/291/5513/2540?ck=nck (accessed July 5, 2008).

Chapter 5
New Discoveries About Fruit and Your Health

1. American Heart Association, "Mediterranean Diet," http://www.americanheart.org/presenter.jhtml?identifier=4644 (accessed July 5, 2008).

2. N. Scarmeas et al., "Mediterranean Diet, Alzheimer's Disease, and Vascular Mediation," *Archives of Neurology* 63 (2006): 1709–1717.

3. D. Qi et al., "Fruit and Vegetable Juices and Alzheimer's Disease: The Kame Project," *American Journal of Medicine* 119, no. 9 (2006): 751–759.

4. L. Azadbakht et al., "Beneficial Effects of Dietary Approach to Stop Hypertension Eating Plan on Features of the Metabolic Syndrome," *Diabetes Care* 28 (2005): 2823–2831.

5. T. Fung et al., "Adherence to a DASH-style Diet and Risk of Coronary Heart Disease and Stroke in Women," *Circulation* 116, no. II (2007): 519.

6. F. J. He, C. A. Nowson, and G. A. MacGregor, "Fruit and Vegetable Consumption and Stroke: Meta-Analysis of Cohort Studies," *Lancet* 367, no. 9507 (2006): 320–326.

7. L. Chatzi et al., "Protective Effect of Fruits, Vegetables, and the Mediterranean Diet on Asthma and Allergies Among Children in Crete," *Thorax* 62 (2007): 677–683.

8. K. T. Khaw et al., "Combined Impact of Health Behaviours and Mortality in Men and Women: The EPIC-Norfolk Prospective Population Study," *PLoS Med* 5, no. 1 (2008): e12.

Chapter 6
Antioxidants = "Anti-Rust" and Phytonutrients

1. Shane Heaton, "Focus on Organic Food Quality—Phytonutrients," *Australian Organic Journal* (Winter 2003): 8–9, http://www.bfa.com.au/_files/AOJ%20Ed%2054_p8-9.pdf (accessed July 23, 2008).

2. Ibid.

3. *Prevention*, "Colors of Health," WedMD.com, http://www.webmd.com/food-recipes/features/colors-health (accessed July 24, 2008).

4. A. G. Schauss et al., "Antioxidant Capacity and Other Bioactivities of the Freeze-dried Amazonian Palm Berry, *Euterpe Oleracea Mart.* (Acai)," *Journal of Agriculture and Food Chemistry* 54, no. 22 (2006): 8604–8610.

5. U.S. Department of Agriculture, "Can Foods Forestall Aging?" http://www.ars.usda.gov/is/AR/archive/Feb99/aging0299.htm (accessed July 24, 2008).

6. TheNibble.com, "A Guide to High-Antioxidant Food," http://thenibble.com/reviews/nutri/overview-of-antioxidants.asp (accessed July 23, 2008).

7. Linda Antinoro, "A Radical Notion: Maybe Antioxidants Can't Protect Us After All," *Environmental Nutrition* (March 2005), viewed at http://findarticles.com/p/articles/mi_m0854/is_3_28/ai_n17212035/pg_2 (accessed July 23, 2008).

8. Christopher Wanjek, "Antioxidants: The Good, the Bad, and the Evil," Mercola.com, http://articles.mercola.com/sites/articles/archive/2001/08/22/antioxidants-part-one.aspx (accessed July 23, 2008).

9. Ibid.

10. CRN.org, "CRN Launches Campaign to Reassure Public of Vitamin E Safety and Benefits," Council for Responsible Nutrition press release, November 29, 2004, http://www.vitamine-index.com/VitaminE/pdfs/CRNPressReleaseNov29.pdf (accessed July 23, 2008).

11. T. Morinobu et al., "The Safety of High-Dose Vitamin E Supplementation in Healthy Japanese Male Adults," *J Nutr Sci Vitaminol* (Tokyo) 48, no. 1 (February 2002): 6–9, http://www.ncbi.nlm.nih.gov/pubmed/12026191?dopt=abstract (accessed July 23, 2008).

12. H. Kappus and A. T. Diplock, "Tolerance and Safety of Vitamin E: A Toxicological Position Report," *Free Radic Biol Med* 13, No. 1 (1992): 55–74, http://www.ncbi.nlm.nih.gov/pubmed/1628854 (accessed July 23, 2008).

13. Earl S. Ford, Umed A. Ajani, and Ali H. Mokdad, "Brief Communication: The Prevalence of High Intake of Vitamin E From the Use of Supplements Among U.S. Adults," *Annals of Internal Medicine* 143, no. 2 (July 19, 2005): 116–120, http://www.annals.org/cgi/content/full/143/2/116 (accessed July 23, 2008).

14. DrWeil.com, "Q & A Library: Should Women Give Up Vitamin E?" August 9, 2005, http://www.drweil.com/drw/u/id/QAA356880 (accessed July 23, 2008).

15. HSIBaltimore.com, "Effects of Vitamin E on Patients With Mild Cognitive Impairment," April 20, 2005, http://www.hsibaltimore.com/ealerts/ea200504/ea20050420.html (accessed July 23, 2008).

16. Ibid.

17. Canadian Asthma Prevention Institute, "Rebuttal to Recent JAMA Reported Study," http://www.asthmaworld.org/vitaminestudy.htm (accessed July 23, 2008).

18. The Healthier Life, "Vitamin E: Another Media Misrepresentation of Vitamin E," August 15, 2005, http://www.thehealthierlife.co.uk/natural-remedies/vitamins/media-misrepresentation-vitamin-e-00404.html (accessed July 23, 2008).

19. Go Ask Alice, "Beta-carotene," May 31, 1996, http://www.goaskalice.columbia.edu/0926.html (accessed July 23, 2008).

Chapter 7
The 411 on Fruits

1. Stephen Cherniske, MSc, "The Acid/Alkaline Mystery Solved," AgingHealthier.com, http://www.aginghealthier.com/pdfs/AcidAlkaline MysterySolved.pdf (accessed July 15, 2008).

2. Ibid.

3. Ibid.

4. Ibid.

5. Ibid.

6. Ibid.

7. R. S. S. Murrieta, D. L. Dufour, and A. D. Siqueira, "Food Consumption and Subsistence in Three Cabaclo Populations on Marajo Island, Amazonia, Brazil," *Human Ecology* 27 (1999): 455–475.

8. A. G. Schauss et al. "Phytochemical and Nutrient Composition of the Freeze-dried Amazonian Palmberry, *Euterpe Oleracea Mart.* (Acai)," *Journal of Agriculture and Food Chemistry* 54, no. 22 (2006): 8598–8603.

9. *Marines*, "Step on a Crack…: Marine Corps Superstitions," April–June 2006, http://www.mcnews.info/mcnewsinfo/marines/2006/20062nd/divisions/pme.shtml (accessed July 23, 2008).

10. Copperwiki.org, "Apricot," http://www.copperwiki.org/index.php/Apricot (accessed July 23, 2008).

11. D. Ruiz et al., "Phytonutrient Content in New Apricot (*Prunus Armeniaca L.*) Varieties," in F. Romojaro, F. Dicenta, and P. Martinez-Gomez, eds., *Proceedings of the Thirteenth International Symposium on Apricot Breeding and Culture* (Muricia, Spain: Acta Horticulturae, n.d.), 363–368.

12. X. Wu et al., "Characterization of Anthocyanins and Proanthocyanins in Some Cultivars of Ribes, Aronia and Sambucus and Their Antioxidant Capacity," *Journal of Agriculture and Food Chemistry* 52 (2004): 846–856.

13. Raintree Nutrition, "Topical Plant Database: Camu Camu," http://www.rain-tree.com/camu.htm (accessed July 23, 2008).

14. AsiaOne.com, "The Kiwifruit Is From China. Right or Wrong?" March 19, 2008, http://www.asiaone.com/Wine%252CDine+%2526+Unwind/News/Food+%2526+Wine/Story/A1Story20080319-55308.html (accessed July 23, 2008).

15. JewishRecipes.org, "Spices and Ingredients: Pomegranate," http://www.jewishrecipes.org/spices/pomegranate.html (accessed July 23, 2008).

Chapter 8
The Three Fs—Fiber, Fructose, and Fruit Juice

1. J. Anderson and S. Perryman, "Dietary Fiber," Colorado State University Extension, May 2007, http://www.ext.colostate.edu/pubs/foodnut/09333.html (accessed July 23, 2008).

2. V. L. Fulgoni III, S. A. Fulgoni, and S. K. Taylor, "Consumption of 100% Juices Is Not Associated With Being Overweight or Risk for Being Overweight in Children," paper presented at the meeting of the Federation of American Societies for Experimental Biology, San Francisco, CA, April 2006.

3. Qi et al., "Fruit and Vegetable Juices and Alzheimer's Disease: The Kame Project."

4. Ruxton, Gardner, and Walker, "Can Pure Fruit and Vegetable Juices Protect Against Cancer and Cardiovascular Disease Too? A Review of the Evidence."

5. Ibid., 15–16.

6. Ibid., 15.

7. Ibid., 19.

Chapter 9
The Quest for Better Health

1. Centers for Disease Prevention and Control, "Heart Disease," http://www.cdc.gov/heartdisease/ (accessed July 14, 2008).

2. World Heart Federation, "Diet," http://www.world-heart-federation.org/cardiovascular-health/cardiovascular-disease-risk-factors/diet (accessed July 23, 2008).

3. Laura Yochum et al., "Dietary Flavonoid Intake and Risk of Cardiovascular Disease in Post Menopausal Women," *American Journal of Epdemiology* 149, no. 10 (May 15, 1999): 943–949.

4. National Center for Health Statistics, "Deaths—Leading Causes," http://www.cdc.gov/nchs/fastats/lcod.htm (accessed July 14, 2008).

5. As referenced in MedicalNewsToday.com, "Antioxidant-rich Diets Reduce Brain Damage From Stroke in Rats," *Medical News Today*, April 13, 2005, http://www.medicalnewstoday.com/articles/22718.php (accessed July 23, 2008).

6. Andis Robeznieks, "Doctors Warned on Single High Blood Pressure Reading," AMedNews.com, August 16, 2004, http://ama-assn.org/amednews/2004/08/16/prsd0816.htm (accessed July 23, 2008).

7. Jeanie Lerche Davis, "Fruits and Veggies Lower Blood Pressure," WebMD .com, May 28, 2002, http://www.webmd.com/diet/news/20020528/fruits-veggies -lower-blood-pressure (accessed July 23, 2008).

8. Hsiang-Ching Kung, PhD, et al., "Deaths: Final Data for 2005," *National Vital Statistics Report* 56, no. 10 (April 24, 2008): http://www.cdc.gov/nchs/data/ nvsr/nvsr56/nvsr56_10.pdf (accessed July 12, 2008).

9. Liz Szabo, "Plant Foods to the Rescue," USAToday.com, August 10, 2004, http://www.usatoday.com/news/health/2004-08-10-plant-foods_x.htm (accessed July 23, 2008).

10. National Center for Health Statistics, "Monitoring Health Care in America: Quarterly Fact Sheet, December 1996," http://www.cdc.gov/nchs/pressroom/ 96facts/mhc1296.htm (accessed July 23, 2008).

11. I. Miedema et al., "Dietary Determinants of Long-term Incidence of Chronic Nonspecific Lung Diseases: The Zutphen Study," *American Journal of Epidermiology* 138 (1993): 37–45.

12. Anthony Wilson, "Carotenoids in Fruits and Vegetables May Cut Arthritis Risk," Arthritis News, Articles, and Information, March 12, 2008, http://www .healthhubs.net/arthritis/carotenoids-in-fruits-vegetables-may-cut-arthritis-risk (accessed July 23, 2008).

13. M. A. Van Duyn at al., "Overview of the Health Benefits of Fruit and Vegetable Consumption," *Journal of the American Dietetic Association* 100 (2000): 1511.

14. Szabo, "Plant Foods to the Rescue."

15. Susan E. Gebhardt and Robin G. Thomas, *Nutritive Value of Foods*, Home and Garden Bulletin Number 72, U.S. Department of Agriculture, http://www .nal.usda.gov/fnic/foodcomp/Data/HG72/hg72_2002.pdf (accessed July 12, 2008).

16. Glenn Barnett, "The Blood of Nelson," *Military History*, October 2006, as quoted in "Grog," http://www.grog.eu/ (accessed July 13, 2008).

17. W. Lee Cowden et al., *Longevity* (Tiburan, CA: n.p., 2001), 142–145.

18. U.S. Department of Agriculture, Agriculture Research Service, "What We Eat in America, NHANES," http://www.ars.usda.gov/Services/docs.htm?docid =15044 (accessed July 23, 2008).

19. BioMedicine.org, "High Vitamin A Increases Risk of Hip Fractures," http:// www.bio-medicine.org/medicine-news/high-vitamin-a-increases-risk-of-hip -fractures-879-1/ (accessed July 23, 2008).

20. National Cancer Institute, "Alpha-Tocopherol, Beta-Carotene Cancer Prevention Trial," July 22, 2003, http://www.cancer.gov/newscenter/pressreleases/ ATBCfollowup (accessed July 24, 2008).

21. Bonnie Liebman, "Antioxidants Report Sets Ceilings," *Nutrition Action Newsletter*, June 2000, http://findarticles.com/p/articles/mi_m0813/is_5_27/ai_ 62494971 (accessed July 24, 2008).

22. UCLA School of Public Health, "Live Longer With Vitamin C," *Newsweek*, May 18, 1992, http://www.newsweek.com/id/125793 (accessed July 24, 2008).

23. Alexandra K. Adams, Ellen O. Wermuth, and Patrick E. McBride, "Antioxidant Vitamins and the Prevention of Coronary Heart Disease," *American Family Physician*, September 1, 1999, http://findarticles.com/p/articles/mi_m3225/ is_3_60/ai_56959011 (accessed July 24, 2008).

24. Jeanie Lerche Davis, "Vitamin C Protects Against Cataracts," WebMD .com, February 22, 2002, http://www.webmd.com/content/Article/24/1738_52446 .htm (accessed July 24, 2008).

25. Anthony J. Brown, MD, "Vitamin C Protects Against Rheumatoid Arthritis," http://www.advancedhealthplan.com/bharthritis.html (accessed July 24, 2008).

26. Heath Davis Havlik, "Overcoming Lupus Fatigue, Naturally," *Better Nutrition*, January 2000, http://findarticles.com/p/articles/mi_m0FKA/is_1_62/ ai_61397507 (accessed July 24, 2008).

27. Centers for Disease Control, "Use of Supplements Containing Folic Acid Among Women of Childbearing Age—United States, 2007," *Morbidity and Mortality Weekly Report*, synopsis for January 10, 2008, http://www.cdc.gov/ media/mmwrnews/2008/n080110.htm#1 (accessed July 24, 2008).

28. John P. Forman et al., "Folate Intake and the Risk of Incident Hypertension Among US Women," *Journal of the American Medical Association* 293, no. 3 (January 19, 2005): 320–329, http://jama.ama-assn.org/cgi/content/ abstract/293/3/320 (accessed July 24, 2008).

29. DNC.com, "Folic Acid May Keep Seniors Sharper," Daily News Central, June 21, 2005, http://health.dailynewscentral.com/content/view/1103/ (accessed July 24, 2008).

30. Linda Brookes, "NORVIT: The Norwegian Vitamin Trial," MedscapeToday .com, http://www.medscape.com/viewarticle/512905 (accessed July 24, 2008).

31. Cowden et al., *Longevity*, 139–141.

32. Jeffrey Blumberg, "Vitamins and Minerals," *Nutrition Action Newsletter*, January/February 2003.

33. Saccharin.org, "History of Saccharin," http://www.saccharin.org/history .html (accessed July 13, 2008).

34. Michelle Meadows, "Healthier Eating," *FDA Consumer Magazine*, May–June 2005, http://www.fda.gov/fdac/features/2005/305_eat.html#lowersodium (accessed July 24, 2008).

35. Elzbieta M. Kurowska et al., "HDL-Cholesterol-Raising Effect of Orange Juice in Subjects With Hypercholesterolemia," *American Journal of Clinical Nutrition* 72, no. 5 (November 2000): 1095–1100, http://www.ajcn.org/cgi/content/ full/72/5/1095 (accessed July 24, 2008).

36. Salynn Boyles, "Noni Juice: Can It Lower Cholesterol?" WebMD.com, March 2, 2006, http://www.webmd.com/cholesterol-management/news/20060302/ noni-juice-can-lower-cholesterol (accessed July 24, 2008).

Chapter 10
Wild, Organic, or Chemical—Does It Really Matter?

1. Catherine Green and Carolyn Dimitri, "Organic Agriculture: Gaining Ground," *AmberWaves*, February 2003, http://www.ers.usda.gov/amberwaves/ feb03/findings/organicagriculture.htm (accessed July 24, 2008).

2. OrganicMonitor.com, "North America Fuelling Global Market Expansion," *The Global Market for Organic Food & Drink*, #7001-40, July 2003, http://www .organicmonitor.com/700140.htm (accessed July 13, 2008).

3. OrganicMonitor.com, "Global Sales of Organic Food & Drink Approaching $40 Billion," *The Global Market for Organic Food & Drink*, #7002-40, http://www. organicmonitor.com/700240.htm (accessed July 13, 2008).

4. U.S. Department of Agriculture, "Labeling Packaged Products," http://www .ams.usda.gov/AMSv1.0/getfile?dDocName=STELDEV3004323&acct=nopgeninfo (accessed July 13, 2008).

5. As quoted in Dave Juday, "Are Organic Foods Really Better for You?" Center for Global Food Issues, February 11, 2000, http://www.cgfi.org/2000/02/11/are -organic-foods-really-better-for-you/ (accessed July 13, 2008).

6. Center for Food Safety and Applied Nutrition, "Pesticide Program Residue Monitoring 2003," May 2005, http://www.cfsan.fda.gov/~dms/pes03rep.html (accessed July 24, 2008).

7. Brian P. Baker et al., "Pesticide Residues in Conventional, IPM-grown and Organic Foods: Insights From Three U.S. Data Sets," *Food Additives and Contaminants* 19, no. 5 (May 2002): 427–446, viewed at http://www .consumersunion.org/food/organicsumm.htm (accessed July 13, 2008).

8. Virginia Worthington, "Effect of Agricultural Methods on Nutritional Quality: A Comparison of Organic With Conventional Crops," *Alternative Therapies* 4 (1998): 58–69, reported in "The Case for Organics: Scientific Studies and Reports," http://journeytoforever.org/garden_organiccase.html (accessed July 24, 2008).

Chapter 11
How Do I Know I'm Getting Enough Fruit?

1. American Optometric Association, "Lutein and Zeaxanthin—Eye-Friendly Nutrients," http://www.aoa.org/x4732.xml (accessed July 25, 2008).

2. Office of Dietary Supplements, "Dietary Supplement Fact Sheet: Vitamin A and Carotenoids," National Institutes of Health, http://ods.od.nih.gov/factsheets/vitamina.asp (accessed July 25, 2008).

3. Ibid.

4. B. Olmedilla et al., "Serum Status of Carotenoids and Tocopherols in Patients With Age-Related Cataracts: A Case-Control Study," *Journal of Nutritional Health Aging* 6, no. 1 (2002): 66–68. F. Khachik et al., "The Effect of Lutein and Zeaxanthin Supplementaion on Metabolites of These Carotenoids in the Serum of Persons Aged 60 or Older," *Invest Ophthamol Vis Sci* 47, no. 12 (December 2006): 5234–5242.

5. Jeanelle Boyer and Rui Hai Liu, "Apple Phytochemicals and Their Health Benefits," *Nutrition Journal* 3, no. 5 (2004): http://www.nutritionj.com/content/3/1/5 (accessed July 25, 2008).

Conclusion
Super Fruits—Myth, Miracle, or Malarkey?

1. Lidija Jakobek et al., "Antioxidant Activity and Polyphenols of Aronia in Comparison to Other Berry Species," *Agriculturae Conspectus Scientificus* 72, no. 4 (2007): 301–306, http://www.agr.hr/smotra/pdf_72/acs72_49.pdf (accessed July 25, 2008).

2. Murrieta, Dufour, and Siqueira, "Food Consumption and Subsistence in Three Caboclo Populations on Marajo Island, Amazonia, Brazil."

3. For example, Schauss et al., "Antioxidant Capacity and Other Bioactivities of the Freeze-dried Amazonian Palm Berry, *Euterpe Oleracea Mart.* (Acai)."

4. Schauss et al. "Phytochemical and Nutrient Composition of the Freeze-dried Amazonian Palmberry, *Euterpe Oleracea Mart.* (Acai)."

Selected Bibliography

Antinoro, Linda. "A Radical Notion: Maybe Antioxidants Can't Protect Us After All." *Environmental Nutrition* (March 2005).

Azadbakht, L., P. Mirmiran, A. Esmaillzadeh, T. Azizi, and F. Azizi. "Beneficial Effects of Dietary Approach to Stop Hypertension Eating Plan on Features of the Metabolic Syndrome." *Diabetes Care* 28 (2005).

Basiotis, P. P., P. Lino, and J. M. Dinkins. "Consumption of Food Group Servings: People's Perceptions vs. Reality." *Nutrition Insights* 20 (2000).

Blanck, H. M., D. A. Galuska, C. Gillespie, L. K. Khan, M. K. Serdula, M. K. Solera, A. H. Mokdad, and L. P. Cohen. "Fruit and Vegetable Consumption Among Adults—United States, 2005." *Morbidity and Mortality Weekly Report* 56, no. 10 (2007).

Chatzi, L., G. Apostolaki, I. Bibakis, I. Skypala, V. Bibaki-Liakou, N. Tzanakis, M. Kogevinas, and P. Cullinan. "Protective Effect of Fruits, Vegetables and the Mediterranean Diet on Asthma and Allergies Among Children in Crete." *Thorax* 62 (2007).

Danaei, G., S. Vander Hoorn, A. D. Lopez, C. J. L. Murray, and M. Ezzati. "Causes of Cancer in the World: Comparative Risk Assessment of Nine Behavioural and Environmental Risk Factors." *Lancet* 366, no. 9499 (2005).

Ello-Martin, J. A., L. S. Roe, J. H. Ledikwe, A. M. Beach, and B. J. Rolls. "Dietary Energy Density in the Treatment of Obesity: A Year-Long Trial Comparing 2 Weight-Loss Diets." *American Journal of Nutrition* 85, no. 6 (2007).

Ford, Earl S., Umed A. Ajani, and Ali H. Mokdad. "Brief Communication: The Prevalence of High Intake of Vitamin E From the Use of Supplements Among U.S. Adults." *Annals of Internal Medicine* 143, no. 2 (July 19, 2005).

Fulgoni, V. L. III, S. A. Fulgoni, and S. K. Taylor. "Consumption of 100 Percent Juices Is Not Associated With Being Overweight or Risk for Being Overweight in Children." Paper presented at the meeting of the Federation of American Societies for Experimental Biology, San Francisco, CA, April 2006.

Fung, T., S. Chiuve, M. McCullough, K. Rexrode, and F. Hu. "Adherence to a DASH-style Diet and Risk of Coronary Heart Disease and Stroke in Women." *Circulation* 116, no. II.

He, F. J., C. A. Nowson, and G. A. MacGregor. "Fruit and Vegetable Consumption and Stroke: Meta-analysis of Cohort Studies." *Lancet* 367, no. 9507 (2006).

Kappus, H. and A. T. Diplock. "Tolerance and Safety of Vitamin E: A Toxicological Position Report." *Free Radic Biol Med* 13, No. 1 (1992).

Khachik, F. et al., "The Effect of Lutein and Zeaxanthin Supplementaion on Metabolites of These Carotenoids in the Serum of Persons Aged 60 or Older." *Invest Ophthamol* Vis Sci 47, no. 12 (December 2006).

Khaw, K. T., N. Wareham, S. Bingham, A. Welch, R. Luben, and N. Day. "Combined Impact of Health Behaviours and Mortality in Men and Women: The EPIC-Norfolk Prospective Population Study." *PLoS Med* 5, no. 1 (2008).

Kurowska, Elzbieta M. et al. "HDL-Cholesterol-Raising Effect of Orange Juice in Subjects With Hypercholesterolemia." *American Journal of Clinical Nutrition* 72, no. 5 (November 2000).

Lewis, C. J. et al. "Nutrient Intakes and Body Weights of Persons Consuming High and Moderate Levels of Added Sugars." *Journal of the American Dietetic Association* 92 (1992).

Miedema, I. et al. "Dietary Determinants of Long-term Incidence of Chronic Nonspecific Lung Diseases: The Zutphen Study." *American Journal of Epidermiology* 138 (1993).

Morinobu, T. et al. "The Safety of High-Dose Vitamin E Supplementation in Healthy Japanese Male Adults." *J Nutr Sci Vitaminol* (Tokyo) 48, no. 1 (February 2002).

Murrieta, R. S. S., D. L. Dufour, and A. D. Siqueira. "Food Consumption and Subsistence in Three Caboclo Populations on Marajo Island, Amazonia, Brazil." *Human Ecology* 27 (1999).

Olmedilla, B. et al., "Serum Status of Carotenoids and Tocopherols in Patients With Age-Related Cataracts: A Case-Control Study." *Journal of Nutritional Health Aging* 6, no. 1 (2002).

Qi, D., A. R. Borenstein, Y. Wu, J. C. Jackson, and E. B. Larson. "Fruit and Vegetable Juices and Alzheimer's Disease: The Kame Project." *American Journal of Medicine* 119, no. 9 (2006).

Ridker, P. M. "Clinical Application of C-reactive Protein for Cardiovascular Disease Detection and Prevention." *Circulation* 107 (2003).

Rinn, Roger C. and Allan Markle. *Positive Parenting*. N.p.: Research Media, 1977.

Ruiz, D., J. Egea, M. I. Gil, and F. A. Tomas-Barberan. "Phytonutrient Content in New Apricot (*Prunus armeniaca L.*) Varieties." (2006). In F. Romojaro, F. Dicenta, and P. Martinez-Gomez, eds., *Proceedings of the Thirteenth International Symposium on Apricot Breeding and Culture*. Muricia, Spain: Acta Horticulturae, n.d.

Ruxton, C. H. S., E. J. Gardner, and D. Walker. "Can Pure Fruit and Vegetable Juices Protect Against Cancer and Cardiovascular Disease Too? A Review of the Evidence." *International Journal of Food Sciences and Nutrition* (2006).

Scarmeas, N., Y. Stern, R. Mayeax, and J. A. Luchsinger. "Mediterranean Diet, Alzheimer's Disease, and Vascular Mediation." *Archives of Neurology* 63 (2006).

Schauss, A. G., X. Wu, R. L. Prior, B. Ou, D. Huang, J. Owens, A. Agarwal, G. S. Jensen, A. N. Hart, and E. Shanbrom. "Antioxidant Capacity and Other Bioactivities of the Freeze-Dried Amazonian Palm Berry, *Euterpe Oleracea Mart.* (Acai)." *Journal of Agriculture and Food Chemistry* 54, no. 22 (2006).

Schauss, A. G., X. Wu, R. L. Prior, B. Ou, D. Patel, D. Huang, and J. P. Kababick. "Phytochemical and Nutrient Composition of the Freeze-dried Amazonian Palmberry, *Euterpe Oleracea Mart.* (Acai). *Journal of Agriculture and Food Chemistry* 54, no. 22 (2006).

Sears, Barry. *Omega Rx Zone.* New York: Harper, 2004.

Seligman, Martin E. P. et al. *Learned Helplessness.* N.p.: Oxford University Press USA, 1995.

Seligman, Martin E. P. *Learned Optimism.* N.p.: Vintage, 2006.

Van Duyn, M. A. et al. "Overview of the Health Benefits of Fruit and Vegetable Consumption." *Journal of the American Dietetic Association* 100 (2000).

Walston, J., M. A. McBurnie, A. Newman, R. P. Tracy, W. J. Kip, C. H. Hirsch, J. Gottdiener, and L. P. Fried. "Frailty and Activation of the Inflammation and Coagulation Systems With and Without Clinical Comorbidities." *Archives of Internal Medicine* 162 (2002).

Wu, X., L. Gu, R. L. Prior, S. McKay. "Characterization of Anthocyanins and Proanthocyanins in some Cultivars of *Ribes*, *Aronia* and *Sambucus* and Their Antioxidant Capacity." *Journal of Agriculture and Food Chemistry* 52 (2004).

Yochum, Laura et al. "Dietary Flavonoid Intake and Risk of Cardiovascular Disease in Post Menopausal Women." *American Journal of Epdemiology* 149, no. 10 (May 15, 1999).